Radiology
for dental auxiliaries

Radiology for dental auxiliaries

HERBERT H. FROMMER, A.B., D.D.S.

Associate Professor and Director of Radiology
New York University College of Dentistry
New York City

Diplomate of the American Board of Oral and Maxillofacial Radiology

FIFTH EDITION

with 456 illustrations

**M Mosby
Year Book**

St. Louis   Baltimore   Boston   Chicago   London   Philadelphia   Sydney   Toronto

Mosby
Year Book

Dedicated to Publishing Excellence

Editor: Robert W. Reinhardt
Assistant Editor: Melba Steube
Project Supervisor: Barbara Bowes Merritt

FIFTH EDITION

Previous editions copyrighted 1974, 1978, 1983, 1987

Printed in the United States of America

Library of Congress Cataloging-in-Publication Data

Frommer, Herbert H.

    Radiology for dental auxiliaries / Herbert H. Frommer. — 5th ed.
      p. cm.

    Includes bibliographical references and index.
    ISBN 0-8016-1701-4
    1. Teeth—Radiography. 2. Dental assistants. I. Title.
    [DNLM: 1. Dental Auxiliaries. 2. Radiography, Dental. WN 230
F932r]
RK309.F76 1992
617.6′07572′024613—dc20
DNLM/DLC   91-15497
for Library of Congress   CIP

C/MV 9 8 7 6 5 4 3 2 1

Preface

It is now 17 years since the first edition of this text was published in 1974. I have been very gratified by the continued response and support of the profession for this book. It has motivated me to try to make each ensuing edition superior to its predecessors. Through the years I have attempted to keep up with and respond to the changes in dentistry and the field of radiology in particular.

The aim of this edition is the same as in the previous four editions: to present the basic principles of radiation physics, radiation biology, protection, technique, and diagnosis in a straightforward and readily understandable manner so those preparing for careers as dental auxiliaries can achieve clinical competency. This clinical competency will then be based on knowledge and understanding and not performed by rote or in a cookbook fashion.

This edition has new chapters on infection control, panoramic radiography, and legal considerations; self-study and examination questions have also been added. Panoramic radiography has become such a large part of dental radiography that a separate chapter is now required. The chapters on infection control and legal considerations reflect current practices in dentistry. My colleagues and friends Dr. Milton Palat, for Legal Considerations, and Dr. Joan Phalen, for Infection Control, deserve special mention for their help in preparing these new chapters. I am also indebted to users of the previous editions for their suggestions and constructive criticisms.

Finally, some words of credit and thanks to some of the people who helped and encouraged me in preparing this fifth edition: to my colleagues in the Radiology Department of the New York University College of Dentistry, Rajinder Jain, Frederick Rich, and Stanley Gibbs; our Dean, Edward G. Kaufman, for creating an atmosphere at the College that encourages scholarship; Carol Robson for her illustrations; and my wife Eleanor and my family for their patience, encouragement, and understanding.

Herbert H. Frommer

To my mother
Ethel Frommer

Contents

Radiology
for dental auxiliaries

1

Ionizing radiation and basic principles of x-ray generation

A preliminary understanding of x-rays and x-ray generation can be acquired by simply visualizing the everyday office procedure of taking a radiograph of a patient. The patient is seated in the dental chair and draped with a lead apron, and a film packet in a film-holding device is positioned in the mouth. The dental x-ray machine (Fig. 1-1) had been previously turned on by an activating switch. The open-ended, rectangular, position-indicating device is then aimed at the film packet in the patient's mouth. The film is exposed by pressing a button attached to an electric cord leading to the x-ray machine. The film is then processed and interpreted by the dentist.

Fig. 1-1. Dental x-ray machine. *A,* Position Indicating Device; *B,* Yoke; *C,* Arm; *D,* Tube head; *E,* Control panel. (Courtesy: Gendex Corp. Milwaukee, Wis.)

From this description, some important observations on the properties of x-rays can be made. X-rays are produced by a machine whose source of energy is electricity; x-rays are produced by pushing a button that completes an electric circuit. Since during the interval of exposure no sign of x-ray production is apparent, it is established that x-rays are invisible. The x-ray beam is directed at the film packet, so x-rays must travel in straight lines.

The ability of x-rays to produce an image on the film packet inside the patient's mouth by a machine positioned outside the mouth indicates that x-rays can penetrate an opaque structure such as skin or teeth.

After having penetrated the dense tissue, x-rays can produce an effect on a photographic emulsion such as the dental film placed in the patient's mouth. This effect is then made visible by processing the film in the darkroom so that an image of the penetrated structures appears on the film.

Because there are undesirable effects from x-rays, the patient is draped with a lead apron for protection and the operator either leaves the room or stands 6 feet away from the machine or behind a suitable barrier when the exposure is made.

In summary, the following are some of the properties of x-rays we have observed:

1. X-rays are produced by the conversion of electric energy into radiation.
2. X-rays are invisible.
3. X-rays travel in straight lines.
4. X-rays can penetrate opaque tissues and structures.
5. X-rays can affect a photographic emulsion, which after processing will produce a visible image.
6. X-rays can adversely affect living tissue.

HISTORY

The x-ray was discovered in November 1895 by Wilhelm Conrad Roentgen, a professor of physics at the University of Wurzberg in Germany. He was working with a vacuum tube called a Crookes tube, through which an electric current was passed (Fig. 1-2). Roentgen, like many of his colleagues, was interested in the cathode ray and the type of light produced across a vacuum tube when an electric current was applied. Since he was concerned with light, he was working in a darkened room with black cardboard covering the Crookes tube, and there were many fluorescent plates in his laboratory. Thus the stage was set for one of the most important discoveries that would aid medical and dental science.

One evening while working in his darkened laboratory, Roentgen noticed that one of the fluorescent plates at the far side of the room was glowing. He quickly realized that something coming from the Crookes tube was striking the fluorescent plate and causing it to glow. Since he did not know what it was, he called the phenomenon x-ray, *x* being the algebraic designation for the unknown. By placing various objects in the path of the x-ray beam, he was able to produce images on the screen. He inadvertently placed his hand between the tube and the screen and saw the faint outline of the bones of his hand. He then went on to expose and produce images on photographic plates. Some of the first radiographs that Roentgen took were of his wife Bertha's hand and his shotgun. Thus we see the first medical and industrial use of x-radiation. It is interesting to note how closely the essential parts of Roentgen's tube and the modern day x-ray tube resemble each other. They both are highly exhausted vacuum tubes having an anode and a cathode through which is passed an electrical current.

A

Fig. 1-2. A, Wilhelm Conrad Roentgen (1845–1925), discoverer of x-rays. **B,** Crookes tube, which Roentgen worked with at the time of the discovery of x-rays in 1895.

Electrons
(cathode ray)

X-radiation

B

+

Induction coil

Roentgen presented a paper on his discovery in late December, and in January 1896 Dr. Otto Walkhoff, a dentist in Braunschweig, Germany, made the first dental use of an x-ray, a radiograph of a lower premolar. He used a small glass photographic plate wrapped in black paper and covered with rubber. The exposure time was 25 minutes. Today, for comparable exposure, we would use about $1/10$ second (6 impulses). For his work in the discovery of x-rays, Roentgen was awarded the first Nobel Prize in physics in 1901. For many years, the science of x-ray was called roentgenology. We still use his name today, expressing the units of x-ray exposure in "roentgens."

C. Edmond Kells, a New Orleans dentist, is credited with having taken the first intraoral radiographs in 1896. Other early workers with intraoral radiographs were W.J. Morton and William Rollins. It was Rollins who developed the first dental x-ray unit in 1896.

Many of the early workers with dental x-rays suffered from effects of their work. William Rollins reported burns to the skin of his hands, and C. Edmond Kells, before his death, had three fingers, his hand, and finally his arm amputated. Dr. Kells used a technique called "setting the tube" to adjust the x-ray beam before radiographing patients. He held his hand between the tube and a fluoroscope and adjusted the beam quality until the bones of his hand were seen clearly.

In 1913, William D. Coolidge invented the hot cathode x-ray tube, which is the prototype of x-ray tubes used today. The hot filament provided a variable source of electrons in the tube and eliminated the need for residual gas as a source for ionization in the tube.

It was also in 1913 that the first American dental x-ray machine was manufactured. In 1923 the Victor X-ray Corporation, which later became General Electric X-ray Corporation, introduced a dental x-ray machine with a Coolidge tube in the head of the unit cooled by oil immersion.

The x-rays were produced in Roentgen's vacuum tube because the electric current applied to the tube caused ionization of the gas molecules in the tube. That is, the neutral molecules were broken up into negative ions and positive ions. Because of the difference in electric potential, the negative particles (electrons) were attracted to the positive side of the tube where they collided with the tube wall, and x-rays were produced. Modern dental x-ray tubes employ the same principle with some modifications, the most significant being a higher voltage or difference in potential across the tube and a variable source of electrons (hot filament), plus radiation safety features and cooling devices.

ATOMIC STRUCTURE

To understand x-ray production and the effect of radiation on tissue, we must understand the basic structure of the atom. All matter is made of atoms. An atom is composed of a relatively heavy inner core or nucleus that possesses a positive electric charge and a number of light, negatively charged particles called *electrons* that orbit around the nucleus (Fig. 1-3). The nucleus of an

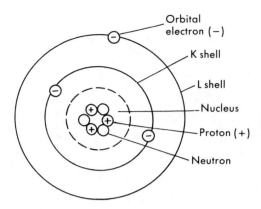

Fig. 1-3. Diagram of an atom. This is a lithium atom whose atomic number (Z) is 3, and its mass number (A) is 6.

atom is composed of positively charged particles called *protons* and particles that have no charge called *neutrons*. The number of protons in the nucleus of an element is specific for each element, determines its atomic number, and is designated by the symbol Z. The total number of protons and neutrons in the nucleus of an atom is the mass number and is designated by the letter *A*. An atom of an element that has the required number of protons but a different number of neutrons in the nucleus is said to be an *isotope* of the element. Isotopes of an element have the same atomic number (number of protons) but a different atomic mass number (number of neutrons) of the element (e.g., carbon-14). They may be stable or unstable, and the unstable isotopes may give off gamma rays. Many isotopes are used as tracer elements in diagnosis or for treatment of malignancies.

In the neutral or stable atom, the number of orbiting electrons (−) equals the number of protons (+) in the nucleus; hence, the atom is electrically neutral.

Electrons travel around the nucleus in definite orbits called *shells*. There is a maximum number of electrons that can occupy each shell and a definite energy level that binds the electrons in each shell to the nucleus. The shells farthest from the nucleus have less binding energy than the inner shells. The shell closest to the nucleus is called the *K shell*, the next outer shell the *L shell*, and then successively the *M, N,* and *O shells*. More energy is needed to remove an electron from the K shell than from the outer shells, because the binding energy is greater.

Atoms in turn join to form molecules. A molecule is the smallest particle of a substance that retains the property of the substance.

IONIZATION

When an orbiting electron is ejected from its shell in an electrically stable or neutral atom, the process is called *ionization* (Fig. 1-4). The electrically neu-

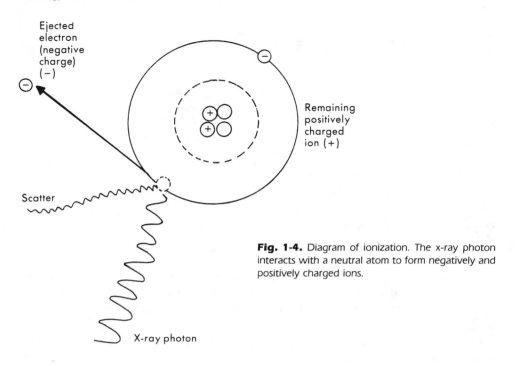

Ejected
electron
(negative
charge)
(−)

Remaining
positively
charged
ion (+)

Scatter

Fig. 1-4. Diagram of ionization. The x-ray photon interacts with a neutral atom to form negatively and positively charged ions.

X-ray photon

tral atom will then be changed into two ions, one positively charged and one negatively. The remainder of the atom has a positive charge, and the ejected electron has a negative charge. Electrons can be removed from atoms by heating or interaction with x-ray photons. In all cases, however, the energy must be greater than the binding energy that holds the electron in orbit around the nucleus of the atom. Thus the inner shell electrons can only be dislodged by high-energy photons such as x-rays, gamma rays, or particulate radiations, while the loosely bound electrons of the outer shell can be dislodged by low-energy photons such as in ultraviolet light. The new ions do not have all the same properties of the former neutral atom. Since x-rays as well as gamma rays and some particulate radiation can cause this type of reaction, they are classified as ionizing radiations. It is the ionizing potential of certain radiations that accounts for their harmful biologic effects. A simple illustration of this is the water molecule, H_2O. If it is ionized, as it can be by radiation, then two hydrogen ions and one oxygen ion are formed. The two ions may recombine to form water again or they may in certain instances recombine as H_2O_2, which is hydrogen peroxide, a tissue poison.

RADIATION

Radiation is the emission and propagation of energy through space or a substance in the form of waves or particles. Particulate radiation consists of atoms or subatomic particles that have mass and travel at high speeds to transmit their kinetic energy. Some examples of particulate radiation are electrons, sometimes called *beta particles*, protons, neutrons, and alpha particles. Particulate radiations most commonly are emitted from radioactive substances called *radionuclides*. Another type of radiation is the wave form. It is with the wave form of radiation that we are most concerned, since x-rays are energy waves with no mass and are part of a grouping called *electromagnetic radiation.*

ELECTROMAGNETIC SPECTRUM

The electromagnetic spectrum is a grouping of energy waves that has in common the weightlessness of the waves and the speed at which they travel (186,000 miles per second). The individual radiations of the spectrum differ in their wavelength and frequency. Those with shorter wavelengths and higher frequency have more photon energy. Looking at Fig. 1-5, we immediately recognize energy waves that we encounter every day.

It is not known whether these electromagnetic radiations are actually waves of energy or the individual units of energy called photons. Some phenomena can be best explained using the wave theory and some by considering the theory of discrete units of energy. If the radiation is considered a wave, it is measured by its length. If it is considered a bundle of photon energy, it can be measured in ergs. We will use both forms in this text, sometimes referring to waves of energy and other to photons of energy.

Let us consider the concept of an energy wave. An energy wave travels in the same way that a ripple crosses a body of still water. The height of the wave is called the crest, and the depth of the wave is called the trough. The distance from one crest to another is called the wavelength and is usually abbreviated with the Greek letter lambda (λ) (Fig. 1-6). The wavelength of x-rays is very short and is measured in Angstrom units, which are $\frac{1}{100,000,000}$ of a centimeter and can be expressed as 10^{-8} cm. The difference in the electromagnetic spectrum between visible light and x-rays is their wavelengths; x-rays have shorter wavelengths. The shorter the wavelength, the more energy it bears, and it is this energy that gives the x-ray the ability to penetrate matter—specifically, the teeth, bones, and gingivae of the dental patient. Light waves cannot penetrate teeth and bone, because the wavelength is too long and thus does not have sufficient energy.

The effect of electromagnetic radiation on living organisms, varies depending on the wavelength. Television waves and radio waves, which are ever present in the atmosphere, have no effect on human tissue. Microwaves, which are low-energy radiations, can produce heat within organic tissues and are so employed in microwave ovens. Microwaves do not have enough energy to be ionizing and therefore do not have the same effects on living tissue as x-rays, gamma rays, or particulate radiations. Electromagnetic radiations that are too low in energy to cause ionization are employed in magnetic resonance imaging (MRI) for diagnostic purposes. These radiations are located in Fig. 1-5 near the radio waves.

Fig. 1-5. Electromagnetic spectrum. The shorter more energized waves to the left are measured in Angstrom units, the longer waves are measured in meters.

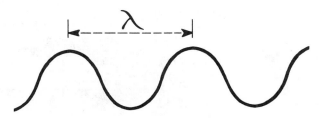

Fig. 1-6. Diagram of x-ray energy wave. The distance between the two crests is the wavelength lambda (λ).

Fig. 1-5 also shows that there is an overlap between gamma rays and the x-rays used for diagnostic purposes in medicine and dentistry, because both have identical wavelengths. Gamma rays and x-rays have identical properties if their wavelengths are the same; they differ only in their source. X-rays are the result of electron and atomic interactions within an x-ray tube, whereas gamma rays originate within the nucleus of radioactive materials.

Ultrasonic radiation is another type of radiation that is used in medicine, and dental patients often question dentists about its use and relationship to dental x-rays. Ultrasound is a nonelectromagnetic, nonionizing radiation that can be used to image internal structures. The fact that it is nonionizing makes its use acceptable in cases in which ionizing radiation might prove harmful (e.g., fetal imaging in pregnant women).

To understand the energy aspect of radiation, let us use the example of throwing a ball. In doing this we are imparting energy to the ball, which is expressed by the speed with which the ball travels. As this energy is lost, the ball falls, hits the ground, and rolls to a stop. The total energy is lost when the ball stops. This is also true of radiation. As x-rays travel over a distance, they lose their energy. For this reason, in the dental office the operator stands a safe distance (6 feet) away from the patient being exposed to x-rays to avoid unnecessary exposure.

If the ball is caught in midair, the energy can be felt by the impact on the hand catching the moving ball. The impact of the ball is in part a product of the weight of the ball and the speed with which it was thrown. X-rays and other radiations have no weight; they have only speed and energy. But their effect is as tangible as the sting of the ball on the hand. This effect is produced by interaction with the basic unit of matter, the atom, and the resultant ionization.

X-RAY PRODUCTION

Radiation is present in our environment coming from the cosmic rays of the sun, radioactive decay of naturally occurring elements, and fallout from manmade sources. For dental and medical purposes, x-rays are produced in an x-ray tube. With modifications, the modern tube resembles the cathode ray tube used by Roentgen, and the principles of high-speed electrons being attracted to

Fig. 1-7. An x-ray tube illustrating formation of an electron cloud at the cathode as filament circuit is activated.

and colliding with a positively charged target to produce x-rays and heat are still valid. Figs. 1-7 through 1-9 are schematic drawings of the production of x-rays in the dental x-ray tube.

When a dental x-ray machine is turned on and the indicator light is glowing, it is ready to produce x-rays. The turning on of the machine completes the filament circuit and heats the tungsten filament in the x-ray tube. The electrons stay at the filament in what is called the "electron cloud" (Fig. 1-7). The electrons will be attracted across the tube only when there is a difference in electric potential or, stated another way, when the high-voltage circuit is completed. This high-voltage circuit is activated by the exposure switch and remains active for the length of time for which a timer is set.

With the high-voltage circuit completed by closing of the exposure switch, the electrons produced by the thermionic emission effect at the cathode are attracted to the positively charged anode, which contains a tungsten target (Fig. 1-8). This stream of electrons crossing the tube is called the *cathode ray*.

Federal regulations require that on new dental x-ray machines an audible signal be sounded when an exposure is being made, in addition to the signal lights in the control panel.[1]

X-rays as well as heat are produced in the tube when the high-speed electrons strike the tungsten target (Fig. 1-9). This is a transference of energy. The kinetic energy of the moving electron is converted into the energy-laden x-ray photon and heat energy. The faster the electrons travel across the tube, the more energized and penetrating will be the x-rays produced. The speed of the electrons across the tube is determined by the kilovoltage.

As illustrated in Fig. 1-15, the tungsten target is angled and the x-rays produced are directed to an exit point (porte) in the tube. The rest of the x-ray tube is lead lined, and it is only through the porte that x-rays can leave the tube. If x-rays leave the tube in any area other than the porte, the machine is said to have head leakage. This is a safety hazard to both patient and operator and a radiation safety code violation.

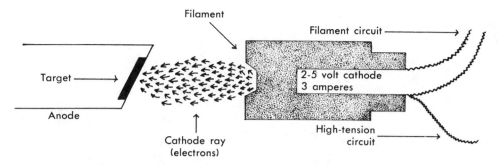

Fig. 1-8. An x-ray tube showing electrons traveling across the tube from the cathode to anode (target) as high-tension circuit (exposure switch) is activated.

Fig. 1-9. An x-ray tube showing production of x-rays as high-speed electrons collide with target.

BREMSSTRAHLUNG AND CHARACTERISTIC X-RAYS

Let us now examine the formation of x-rays at the level of the atom. That is, what is the atomic mechanism of the formation of x-rays when the high-speed electrons strike the tungsten target?

The phenomenon of x-ray production can be best understood by considering the tungsten atom and the possibilities that arise when a high-speed electron enters its orbit, as it would at the target of a dental x-ray machine (Fig. 1-10). The tungsten target is made up of an infinite number of tungsten atoms. We will consider only one surface atom that will serve as a representative example for the rest of the atoms in the tungsten target.

The first possibility, which rarely occurs, is that the high-speed electron might hit the nucleus of the tungsten atom and give up all its energy. The second possibility represented by entering electron A in Fig. 1-10 is that the entering high-speed electron might be slowed down and bent off its course by the positive pull of the nucleus. This slowing down represents a loss of energy that is given off as x-rays and heat. This is the major source of x-ray production in

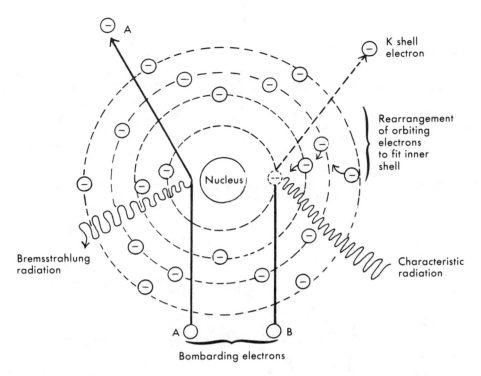

Fig. 1-10. Electrons colliding with a simulated tungsten atom, forming **A,** Bremsstrahlung radiation and **B,** characteristic radiation.

the dental x-ray tube. The slowing down and veering off course of the entering high-speed electron with its loss of energy expressed in x-rays and heat is called *bremsstrahlung,* the German word for "breaking radiation."

Since the tungsten target is not just one atom thick, this bremsstrahlung is repeated an infinite number of times. The exiting electron A' (Fig. 1-10) will enter another tungsten atom, and the reaction will be repeated with the production of more x-rays. A' and the succeeding A", A"', and so forth each will have less energy than the original entering electron A; hence the x-rays produced at each succeeding bremsstrahlung will have less energy or longer wavelengths. Because of the multiple bremsstrahlung reactions, all the x-rays produced do not have the same energy content (wavelength). A heterogeneous x-ray spectrum is produced. The later bremsstrahlung reactions produce x-rays whose energy is not sufficient to penetrate teeth and bone and, as we will see, will be removed by filtration.

The third possibility represented by entering electron B is that the high-speed electron might hit and dislodge one of the orbiting electrons of the tungsten atom. This can happen only when the entering electrons possess more energy than that binding the orbiting electrons to the nucleus. In the dental machine, this means it can happen only at settings of 70 kVp (70,000 volts) and above because the binding energy of the K shell of electrons is 69,000 electron volts. If an orbiting electron is dislodged, there is a rearrangement or cascading of electrons inward to fill up the electron vacancies in the inner shells. This rearrangement produces a loss of energy that is expressed in x-ray energy. The x-rays thus produced are called characteristic x-rays and account for a very small part of the x-rays produced in the dental machine and only in those machines operating at 70 kVp and above.

THE DENTAL X-RAY MACHINE

Electricity

Since the primary source of energy for the x-ray machine is electricity, it is necessary to learn or review some basic concepts of electricity.

Electric current is the flow of electricity through a circuit; it can either be alternating (AC) or direct (DC). By direct current, we mean current that flows in only one direction in an electric circuit, whereas alternating current flows in one direction and then flows in the opposite direction in the circuit (Fig. 1-11). In the dental x-ray tube this means that the tungsten filament is only the negative pole one half the time because of the reversal of the direction of the current. During this part of current flow no x-rays are produced.

The term *cycle* in alternating current refers to the flow of current in one direction and then the reversal and flowing of the current in the opposite direction. There are usually 60 cycles per second in most alternating current circuits.

Rectification. Since the dental x-ray machine is operating on alternating current this means that in the x-ray tube itself the polarity is reversed 60 times per second. When the direction of the current flow is reversed, the tungsten tar-

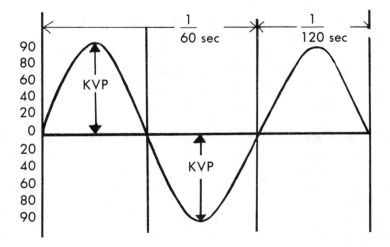

Fig. 1-11. Sine wave of 60-cycle electric current operating at 90,000 volts (90 kVp).

get becomes the negative pole or cathode and the tungsten filament becomes the positive pole or anode. During the alternating $\frac{1}{120}$ second (one-half of a cycle) when the current is reversed, no x-rays are produced, for there are no electrons at the target available to travel across the tube and strike the target, and so the current is blocked from traveling across the tube. This blocking of the reversal is called rectification and since the dental x-ray tube does this because of its own design, it is said to be self-rectified.

X-rays are not produced in a steady stream but in spurts or pulses, and these pulses take place only during one-half of the alternating current cycle. Since most alternating current is 60 cycles, the dental x-ray machines will express exposure units in pulses or sixtieths of a second instead of the usual $\frac{1}{2}$ second or $\frac{3}{10}$ second. A $\frac{1}{2}$-second exposure is equal to 30 pulses. It should be obvious that exposure time of $\frac{1}{7}$ second is not possible, since it is not divisible into 60, and it is impossible to get a fraction of a cycle of alternating current.

Some newer model dental x-ray machines are designed to supply full wave rectification. In this circuitry, the negative portion of the alternating current cycle is reversed. If currents are then superimposed, there is less of a drop in voltage between cycles. These machines do not produce pulses of x-radiation but rather a constant stream of x-rays. Because of this, the exposure time can be reduced by one-half since x-rays are not being produced half the time, as they are in the self-rectified circuit, but all the time. The radiation exposure to the patient is the same, it just takes place in one half the time.

Voltage is the term used to describe the electric potential or force that drives an electric current through a circuit. The unit of measurement is the volt. The kilovolt (kV) is 1000 volts. In an alternating current, where the direction of the current is constantly changing, the voltage is also changing, and the term kilovolt peak (kVp) is used to denote the maximum or peak voltage that is described by the sine wave that plots the alternation of the current (see Fig. 1-11). A dental x-ray machine that is set for a potential of 90 kV will only reach 90 kV at the peak of the alternating current during exposure. As seen in the diagram of the exposure's sine wave, other voltage levels also occur during the exposure. This has great clinical significance, because these differences in voltage contribute to the heterogeneity of the x-ray beam.

Ampere is the unit of measurement used to describe the amount of electric current flowing through a circuit. The milliampere (mA) is equal to $\frac{1}{1000}$ of an ampere.

A *transformer* is a device that can either increase or decrease the voltage in an electric circuit. It is composed of two coils of electric wire insulated from one another. The magnetic field from one coil induces an electric current in the second coil. The number of turns in the induction coil in relation to the number of turns in the second coil will determine what the action of the transformer will be. The dental x-ray machine also has an autotransformer, which utilizes only one coil and can be used only for making minor changes in voltage. If the transformer increases the voltage, it is referred to as a "step-up" transformer, and if it decreases the voltage, it is referred to as a "step-down" transformer. The dental

Fig. 1-12. Diagram of basic electric circuits of dental x-ray machine.

x-ray machine utilizes both types in taking ordinary line or house voltage of 110 volts and stepping it up to a range of 65,000 to 100,000 volts (65 to 100 kVp) in the high-voltage circuit or stepping line voltage down to 3 to 5 volts in the filament circuit, these being the two basic circuits in the dental x-ray machine.

Circuitry

Dental x-ray machines use 110-volt alternating current (Fig. 1-12). There are two major circuits in the x-ray machine, the filament circuit and the high-voltage circuit. Each circuit utilizes a transformer to convert the line voltage and current. The filament circuit uses 3 to 5 volts, and so the 110-volt line current is reduced by means of a step-down transformer. The heating of the cathode filament by the electric current is controlled by a rheostat in the circuit and is a function of the milliamperage selector on the control panel of the machine. The high-voltage circuit in the dental x-ray machine requires voltage in the range of 65,000 to 100,000 volts. This increase in voltage is achieved by the use of a step-up transformer. An auto transformer is also used in the circuit as a line compensator to control fluctuations in line voltage. The relationship of the input circuit to a variable number of coils is changed in the autotransformer, by the kVp dial on the control panel, to change the quality of the x-rays emitted.

Control panel

The control panel of the dental x-ray machine (Fig. 1-13) contains an on-off switch and indicator light, an exposure button and indicator light, timer dial,

Fig. 1-13. Control panel of dental x-ray machine. *A,* Exposure control on a 6-foot retractable cord; *B,* "on" indicator; *C,* exposure indicator; *D,* kVp meter; *E,* kVp control; *F,* mA control; *G,* timer control.

and kVp and mA selectors. The exposure button is on a 6-foot retractable cord or linked to a remote station. Some machines have preset fixed milliamperage choices, usually 7, 10, or 15 mA or adjustable. The kVp values may be fixed or have a range from 65 to 100.

Timer. The dental x-ray tube does not emit a continuous stream of radiation but rather a series of impulses of radiation (Fig. 1-14). The number of impulses depends on the number of cycles per second in the electric current being used. In 60-cycle alternating current, there are 60 pulses of x-ray per second. Each impulse lasts only $\frac{1}{120}$ second, since no x-rays are emitted in the negative half of the cycle when the polarity of the tube is reversed. The newer model dental x-ray machine exposure dials are not calibrated in fractions of seconds, but more realistically in impulses. On the timer dial, "24" means 24 impulses per second, which is equivalent to $\frac{2}{5}$ or $\frac{24}{60}$ second of exposure. With the advent of more sensitive or faster films calling for decreasing exposure times, all machines should have electronically controlled timers so that these short exposure times can be achieved accurately and repeatedly. The old mechanical timers with increments of $\frac{1}{4}$ second, which were usually at least $\frac{1}{8}$ to $\frac{1}{4}$ second inaccurate, are unacceptable for the shorter exposure times in use.

The x-ray machine should be turned off after use. Warm-up time is almost instantaneous for the x-ray tube, so there is no need to keep the machine on during the working day. Most offices will have a definite setting for mA and kVp that is used for all patients. As will be seen in the next chapter, the kVp will be determined by the density of the object and the type of contrast desired, while the mA will be determined by the speed of the film and the exposure time and distance.

The control panel should be checked each day to be sure that the mA and kVp settings have not inadvertently been changed. Some control panels have

Fig. 1-14. Timer dial. Note the increments in impulses (1/60 seconds).

Fig. 1-15. Components of a dental x-ray tube.

preset values for different types of patients, and the selectors are labeled with such terms as "large patient," "child," and so forth. If one understands the principles of radiology, this type of panel is unnecessary and very limiting.

X-ray tube

The dental x-ray tube, housed in a large machine, is about 6 inches long and 1½ inches in diameter.

The three basic elements of an x-ray tube needed to produce x-rays are (1) high voltage to accelerate electrons across the tube, (2) a source of electrons within the tube, and (3) a target to stop the electrons.

High voltage. As shown in Fig. 1-15, the x-ray tube has a positive side (pole) called the anode and a negative side called the cathode. Electric current flows from a negative pole to a positive pole. This voltage can be varied by adjusting the kilovoltage dial that actually controls the autotransformer, which then affects the step-up transformer and thus the kilovoltage across the tube. The greater the kilovoltage or potential across the tube, the faster the electrons will travel and the greater the energy that will be released when the electrons strike the target at the anode.

Source of electrons. The main source of electrons in the x-ray tube is the tungsten filament found at the cathode. This is a variable source of electrons, unlike Roentgen's tube in which electrons were produced from the ionization of a fixed volume of gas. The tungsten filament is connected to the step-down transformer circuit. The hotter the resistant filament becomes, the more electrons that are produced at the cathode. This production, or boiling off, of electrons from the heated tungsten filament is called the thermionic emission effect. The milliamperage dial controls the amount of current in the filament circuit and hence the number of electrons that "boil off." The tungsten filament is surrounded by the molybdenum focusing cup, which directs electrons toward the anode that contains the target.

Target. The target in the x-ray tube can also be called the *focal spot* or area. It is at the anode part of the tube, and when the circuit is complete, it has a positive (+) charge. It is made of tungsten and measures about 0.8 × 1.8 mm. This is the actual target. The effective target or focal area is smaller because of the tilting of the target that geometrically makes the target smaller when viewed from the opening in the tube. All modern dental x-ray machines have approximately the same size target. Tungsten is used as the target material because it has a high melting point and a low vapor pressure at high temperatures and thus will not be affected by the heat produced. The element tungsten is also desirable as a target material because of its high atomic number, and thus its density, and because when it is bombarded by electrons, x-ray production is more efficient. Tungsten, however, does not have a high degree of thermal conductivity and must be imbedded in a copper stem. The heat is dissipated into the head of the x-ray machine by the copper stem attached to the anode and cooled by air or oil immersion.

Heat production. It must be pointed out that the dental x-ray machine is an extremely inefficient machine. That is, of the total energy produced at the anode by the collision of the electrons with the target, less than 1% is x-ray energy; the remaining 99% is in the form of heat. This is the reason for the highly conductive copper sleeve and oil immersion tube surrounding the target. Care must be taken not to overheat the tube.

Heat production is the limiting factor of the mA setting of a dental x-ray machine. With an mA of more than 15 there will be too many electrons hitting the target and too much heat produced. This overheating will soon destroy the target. Some panoramic and extraoral units have rotating anodes to dissipate the heat and thus can use higher mA settings. The standard dental x-ray machine has a fixed anode and thus has a limit to the amount of milliamperage.

Under ordinary use, overheating of a dental x-ray machine is not very likely. Each machine has a duty rating and a duty cycle. The *duty rating* refers to the number of consecutive seconds a machine can be operated before over-heating, and the *duty cycle* refers to the portion of every minute that the dental machine can be used without overheating.

X-RAY BEAM

The x-ray photons produced at the target in the dental x-ray tube emanate from and leave the tube as a divergent beam. The x-ray at the center of the beam is referred to as the central ray. The x-rays closest to the central ray will be more parallel and those farthest away more divergent. It is the more parallel rays that will produce less magnification of the image and the rays that we want to use (Fig. 1-16).

The x-ray beam is positioned or aimed at the film in the patient's mouth by an open-ended device, either a rectangle or a cylinder, called a *position indicating device* (PID). These PIDs should be lead lined to prevent the escape of scatter radiation and are usually 8, 12, or 16 inches in length (Fig. 1-17). Originally, all dental machines had short, 8-inch pointed cones as position indicating devices. To this day, people refer to open-ended cylinders as cones, although the proper term is position indicating device.

The pointed cone was designed as an easy aiming device, the tip of the cone indicating the position of the central ray. The technique called for aiming the tip of the cone at the center of the film packet placed in the patient's mouth or the extraoral anatomic landmark being used. One of the unfortunate out-comes of this type of instrumentation was that some practitioners came to be-lieve that the x-ray beam was coming out only from the tip of the cone and that the size of the beam was that limited.

Fig. 1-16. The divergent x-ray beam. The aluminum filter removes longer wavelength x-rays from the beam.

Fig. 1-17. Position indicating devices, open-ended, lead-lined 8-inch, 12-inch, 16 inch **(A)** rectangles; **(B)** cylinders. (Courtesy Margraf Dental Mfg., Jenkintown, PA.)

The problem with the pointed plastic cone is the secondary radiation that is produced by the interaction of the primary beam of x-ray photons with the plastic cone (Fig. 1-18). These secondary x-rays increase the long wavelength radiation to the patient's face and degrade the diagnostic image on the film. X-rays do interact with plastic, even though one might not consider it to be a very dense material. X-rays will interact and cause secondary radiation with any form of matter from a piece of tissue paper to a bar of steel. The density of the material and the quality of the x-ray beam determine the type and extent of interaction. When the open-ended PID is used, there is no material at the end of the PID with which to interact. Some practitioners have complained about open-ended PIDs, claiming that they are difficult to aim properly and that "cone cutting" results. In reality, it is not that the rectangle or the cylinder is difficult to use but that the change from using the pointed cone is difficult. Novice stu-

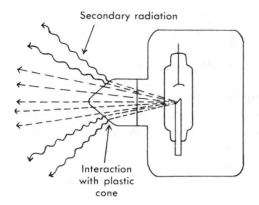

Secondary radiation

Interaction
with plastic
cone

Fig. 1-18. Production of secondary radiation resulting from interaction of the primary beam with the closed-end plastic cone.

dents starting instruction in radiology have no more difficulty using open-ended PIDs than their predecessors had with the pointed one.

Radiation protection codes in many states have mandated the use of the open-ended PIDs. It is strongly recommended that even in jurisdictions that allow the use of pointed cones, their use be terminated and open-ended, lead-lined rectangles or cylinders be used instead. The state of the art in radiation risk prevention calls for open-ended lead-lined PIDs.

Quality and quantity of x-rays: milliamperage and kilovoltage

The three parameters of the dental x-ray beam that are adjusted from the control panel by either the dental auxiliary or the dentist are (1) the energy, or penetrating power (quality), of the x-ray beam, (2) the number of x-rays produced (quantity), and (3) the length of time that these x-rays will be produced.

Quality. The quality, or penetrating power, of the x-ray beam is controlled by the kilovoltage. The suitable range for dental radiography is 65 to 100 kVp. Some units can deliver this complete range, whereas others have more limited ranges or even a fixed kVp value. As a rule, the kilovoltage in a dental office will remain fixed at one setting for all intraoral radiography. The dentist will determine what kilovoltage will produce the most diagnostic radiographs for the particular use of that office.

Dental diagnostic radiology is confined to the 65 to 100 kVp range because the density of the structures dentistry deals with (teeth, bone, etc.) determines the useful penetration range. Kilovoltage settings below 65 would not give proper penetration of the object without undue production of secondary x-radiation, and kilovoltage above 100 causes overpenetration. The overall objective of diagnostic radiology is to record differences in densities on the film of the objects being radiographed. A kilovoltage range is chosen that will indicate the difference of penetration and absorption so that the differences in structural densities can be recorded. The choice of kVp setting will be discussed in the section on density and contrast. We see, then, that a kilovoltage is selected that will allow for complete absorption of some x-rays, partial absorption of others, and passage of other x-rays through the object to reach the film.

The radiograph is produced because of differential absorption of the x-ray beam by the object being radiographed. That is why less dense structures, such as the dental pulp, will appear radiolucent (black) on the dental film, and highly calcified denser structures, such as the enamel, will appear radiopaque (white or gray). The less dense areas in the object allow greater passage of x-rays than do denser areas, and more x-rays strike the film in these areas to darken it.

X-ray machines with a low kilovoltage rating in the 45 to 65 kVp range are no longer considered acceptable, because the radiation produced contains many long, nonpenetrating wavelengths that increase the facial exposure to the patient unnecessarily (see Fig. 4-2).

Half value layer. The term *half value layer* (HVL) is more appropriate than kilovoltage to describe beam quality and penetration. Kilovoltage is a description of the electric energy put into an x-ray tube. HVL measures the quality of the x-rays emitted from the tube. Two similar x-ray machines operating at the same kilovoltage may not produce x-rays of the same penetration. The HVL is defined as the thickness of aluminum (measured in millimeters) that will reduce the intensity of the x-ray beam by 50%. For example, a dental x-ray beam could be described as having an HVL of 2 mm. This would mean that the energy of this particular beam is such that a thickness of 2 mm of aluminum would be necessary to decrease its intensity by half. Another beam having an HVL of 1 mm would not be as energized as only 1 mm of aluminum is necessary to decrease its energy by half.

Quantity. The milliampere dial determines the number of x-rays produced in a given exposure time period by controlling the heating of the tungsten filament at the cathode of the tube. As the kilovoltage determines the quality (penetrating power) of the x-rays produced, the milliamperage determines the quantity of x-rays produced.

It is better to consider the concept of milliampere seconds (mAs) than milliamperage alone. An exposure at a given kVp of 1 second using 10 mA is 10 mAs. A 2-second exposure at the same kVp using 5 mA would produce an identical film, since the mAs are again 10 ($10 \times 1 = 10$, $5 \times 2 = 10$).

The sensitivity of the film and the focal-film distance used determines the mAs required at a given kilovoltage. The more sensitive the film to radiation, the fewer milliampere seconds required. The advantage of higher milliamperage is that a shorter exposure time can be used. This does not represent a decrease in the patient's x-ray exposure, only a decrease in the time necessary to expose the film. This reduces the chance of blurring caused by patient motion.

Ideally, it would be best to use the shortest exposure time and a high milliamperage to achieve the desired mAs. The range of milliamperage on dental x-ray machines is usually from 5 to 15 mA. As previously mentioned, the limiting factor is the heat produced at the desired small target. Milliamperage higher than 15 would produce too many electrons bombarding the target and thus too much heat. Some x-ray machines in dentistry are made specifically for extraoral radiography and have rotating anodes. A rotating anode is a spinning disk composed of many tungsten targets instead of one stationary target, as found in the standard intraoral x-ray unit. Because the targets are rotating, they are struck by the electrons through only part of their 360-degree rotation. During the rest of the rotation, the targets can cool. Since the heat is dissipated in this manner, an mA of 50 or 100 is used.

Filtration. The x-ray beam that originates at the anode is not homogeneous. It consists of a spectrum of long and short wavelengths. In fact, very few of the x-ray photons produced have energy or penetration power corresponding to the desired kilovoltage called for on the control panel. In other words, if one sets the kVp dial for any desired kilovoltage, only a few of the x-ray photons produced will correspond to this setting. Almost all the x-ray photons produced will have wavelengths longer than those corresponding to the desired setting and thus will be less penetrating. This is partially the result of the electrons in the tube bombarding multiple atomic layers of the tungsten target with the resulting bremsstrahlung and characteristic x-ray production and the effect of alternating current with its sine wave voltage buildup. As shown in Fig. 1-19, the x-ray beam is not homogeneous but rather heterogeneous, having a full range of wavelengths. The longer, lower kVp wavelengths will not penetrate tooth and bone and will be absorbed only by the skin or produce secondary radiation.

The function of the filter is to remove from the primary beam the long, nonpenetrating wavelength x-rays (see Fig. 1-16). After the primary beam has been filtered and collimated, it is referred to as the *useful beam.*

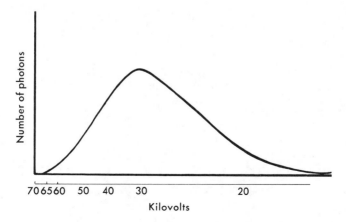

Fig. 1-19. Graph of spectrum of x-ray beam from dental x-ray machine operating at 65 kVp. Note number of low-energy photons produced.

Federal regulations require that for dental x-ray machines operating at kilovoltages up to 70 kVp, 2 mm of aluminum filtration is required.[1] For those machines operating from 70 kVp and higher, 2.5 mm of aluminum filtration is required. All new machines must meet these requirements.

Collimation

The size and shape of the x-ray beam as it leaves the tube head are restricted by a collimating device (Fig. 1-20). In intraoral radiography, the size of the beam should be just large enough to cover the film packet. Circular collimation allows for a slight margin of error in positioning (Fig. 1-21). A beam size any larger than this would expose the patient's face to unnecessary primary radiation. Historically, the diameter of the x-ray beam measured at the patient's

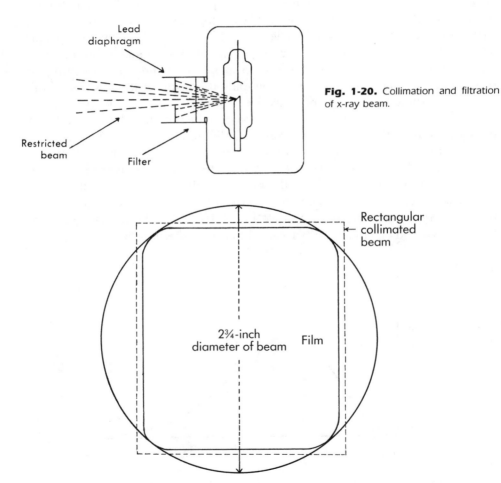

Fig. 1-20. Collimation and filtration of x-ray beam.

Fig. 1-21. Relative size of adult film packet compared to x-ray beam 2¾ inches in diameter and rectangularly collimated beam.

Fig. 1-22. A, Lead diaphragm; B, An aluminum filter.

face used in dentistry has been decreasing. From no limitation at all in the early days of dental radiology, the beam diameter has gone to 3½ inches, 3 inches, and presently is 2¾ inches (7 cm).

The collimating device most often used is a lead diaphragm with a circular aperture (Fig. 1-22). The size of this aperture, at a selected focal-film distance, determines the beam size. PIDs, be they open-ended cylinders or rectangles, lead-lined or made of metal, can also serve as collimating devices. Federal regulations presently require that the x-ray beam should not exceed 2¾ inches (7 cm) in diameter when measured at the patient's skin.[1]

Rectangular collimation. The shape of the dental x-ray beam has always been circular. The question can be asked, "Why is a circular beam used when the film packet is rectangular in shape?" The circular beam covers a greater facial area, and it exposes the patient to more primary radiation than a tightly collimated rectangular beam does. The movement in the dental profession is now toward rectangular collimation. It is being taught as the primary technique in most dental schools and is recommended by the American Dental Association[2] and the American Academy of Oral and Maxillofacial Radiology.[3] This change to rectangular collimation can be accomplished without an increase in "cone cutting" with the use of proper equipment. X-ray beam film alignment is easily done by using the Precision Device (Isaac Masel Co.) (Fig. 1-23), the XCP (Rinn Corp.), and a metal rectangular PID (Fig. 1-24), or many other devices now available. The use of these devices in rectangular collimation is illustrated and described in Chapter 7.

Interaction of x-rays with matter

X-rays interact with all forms of matter. This interaction can result in absorption of energy (a reduction of the intensity of the x-ray beam) and the production of secondary radiation.

Primary radiation is the result of the x-rays produced at the target of the anode in the x-ray tube. Secondary radiation is the result of the interaction of primary radiation with matter (see Fig. 4-1).

Fig. 1-23. Rectangular collimating device. (Courtesy Precision Instruments, Isaac Masel Co., Inc., Philadelphia.)

Fig. 1-24. A, Rectangular PID collimator; **B,** With "XCP."

When x-rays are absorbed by matter, positive and negative ions as well as secondary radiation are formed from previously neutral atoms. The amount and type of absorption that takes place depend on the energy of the x-ray beam (the wavelength) and the composition of the absorbing matter. The thicker the material that an x-ray beam has to penetrate, the more x-rays that will be absorbed. It is, however, not just thickness that determines x-ray absorption. The atomic configuration—the number of orbiting electrons, protons, and neutrons in the nucleus of the atom—also determines x-ray absorption. Heavy elements, those with greater mass, are better absorbers than lighter elements. The more electrons available in an absorbing material, the more x-ray photons that are absorbed. Heavy metals with high atomic numbers (the atomic number indicates the number of protons in the nucleus of the atom), such as lead and gold, absorb x-rays readily.

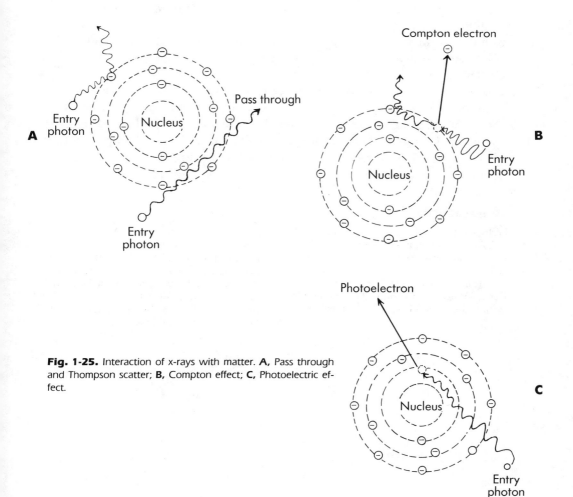

Fig. 1-25. Interaction of x-rays with matter. **A,** Pass through and Thompson scatter; **B,** Compton effect; **C,** Photoelectric effect.

An important point to be made is that when x-rays are absorbed by any material, that material does not become radioactive, because x-rays have no effect on the nucleus of the absorbing atom. This means that the equipment or walls in a dental operatory do not become radioactive after continuous exposure to radiation. At the atomic level, there are four possibilities that can occur when an x-ray photon interacts with matter. These possibilities are:

1. No interaction (pass through). The x-ray photon can pass through the atom unchanged and leave the atom unchanged (Fig. 1-25, A). This will happen about 9% of the time in a bitewing examination.[4]

2. Thompson scatter (unmodified or coherent scatter). In effect the x-ray photon has its path altered by the atom. There is no change to the absorbing atom, but a photon of scattered radiation is produced (Fig. 1-25, A). This accounts for about 8% of the interactions that take place in dental radiography.[4]

3. Photoelectric effect. The x-ray photon can collide with an orbiting electron, giving up all its energy to dislodge the electron from its orbit. The photoelectron that is produced will have a negative charge, while the remaining atom will have a positive charge. This, you will remember, is ionization (Fig. 1-25, C). This interaction takes place about 30% of the time with dental x-rays.[4]

4. Compton effect. The x-ray photon can collide with a loosely bound electron in an outer shell of the atom and only give up part of its energy in ejecting the electron from its orbit. This results in a negatively charged, ejected Compton electron, a photon of scattered radiation, and a remaining atom that is now positively charged. This again is ionization (Fig. 1-25, B). This interaction takes place about 62% of the time in dental x-rays.[4]

REFERENCES

1. Performance standards for electronic products: diagnostic x-ray systems and their major components. Fed Register 37:16461, 1972.

2. American Dental Association, Council on Dental Materials, Instruments, and Equipment: Recommendations in radiographic practices: an update, 1988, J Am Dent Assoc 118:115-117, 1988.

3. American Academy of Oral and Maxillofacial Radiology: Position paper on rectangular collimatiom and E speed film, Oral Surg Oral Med Oral Path (in press).

4. Goaz P and White S: Oral radiology, ed 2, St Louis, 1987, The CV Mosby Co.

2

Image formation, image receptors

FACTORS INFLUENCING IMAGE FORMATION

In making radiographs of dental structures, we are striving for a film image with the proper degree of density and contrast, detail sharpness, and a minimum amount of enlargement and distortion. These factors will enable us to gain the most diagnostic information for the amount of radiation expended.

Density and contrast

Density is the degree of blackness on a film, and contrast is the difference in the degrees of blackness between adjacent areas. The density of a film is determined by the relative transmissions of the x-rays by various parts of the object and by the absorption of the x-rays in the emulsion of the film. These two factors, the object being radiographed (object contrast) and the properties of the film (film contrast) determine the overall density and contrast of the finished radiograph.

Object contrast. The object contrast is determined by (1) the thickness of the object, (2) the density of the object, (3) the chemical composition of the object, (4) the quality of the x-ray beam, and (5) scatter radiation. We cannot control the thickness, density, or atomic number of the structures being radiographed (teeth, bone, etc.), and it is these parameters that determine the range of kVp that is used in dentistry. We are seeking a diferential absorption pattern that will portray differences in object density. Thus using a kVp setting greater than 100 will result in overpenetration and using a kVp of below 45 will conversely result in underpenetration. In both cases the selective penetration desired will not be achieved.

The only variables of object contrast are the quality or penetration of the x-rays within the dental penetration range of 65 to 100 kVp, and the amount of scatter radiation produced.

The image difference between films produced at the different kVp settings in the dental range is the resulting contrast. By varying the kilovoltage and the quality of the radiation, either high- or low-contrast films can be produced.

Short scale. High-contrast films appear mainly black and white with very

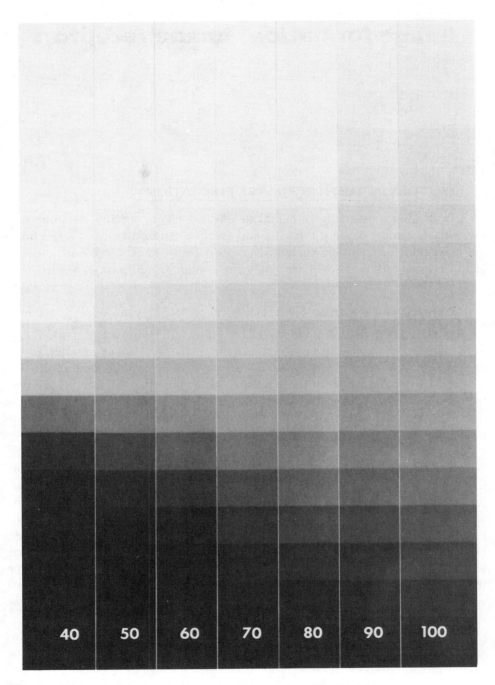

Fig. 2-1. Aluminum step wedge densities. A step wedge of aluminum is radiographed using increasing kVp (penetration). At the thinner portion of the step wedge, there is complete penetration at all kVps. At the thicker portion of the wedge, the lower kVp will not penetrate while the higher kVp will penetrate as shown by the gray tones. (Courtesy Eastman Kodak Co.)

Fig. 2-2. A, High-contrast radiograph taken at 65 kVp. Note predominance of black and white tones. **B,** Low-contrast radiograph taken at 90 kVp. Note predominance of gray tones.

few gray tones. They are also referred to as short-scale contrast films and are produced by kilovoltage in the 55 to 65 kVp range. These films are said to be "crisper" and more pleasing to the eye, but they may not reveal early pathologic changes. The short-scale film is a "yes" or "no" situation: either the x-ray beam penetrates the object or it does not. Areas appear black or white, radiolucent or radiopaque, with few gray tones in the middle range (Figs. 2-1 and 2-2). The lower kVp ratings (below 65) are undesirable because they result in increased facial absorption and scatter as a result of their less-penetrating wavelengths.

Long scale. The low-contrast films, also referred to as long-scale contrast, are produced by the high kilovoltage range of 90 to 100 kVp. In these films, there are many tones of gray in addition to the blacks and whites. The long-scale film is not as visually pleasing as the short-scale film, but early changes in object density may be seen in the gradation of the gray tones, which are not present in the high-contrast films. One could choose a kVp in the middle range (70 to 75 kVp) and try to gain some advantage from both techniques.

Scattered radiation, besides its effect on other parts of the patient's body, produces a uniform exposure or darkening over the film and in doing so reduces the contrast. Scattered radiation is one of the causes of "film fog," and it degrades the diagnostic image. Most scattered radiation originates in the object itself; thus the larger the field, the more that scatter becomes a factor. As we will see in Chapter 9, grids are sometimes used to eliminate object scatter in extraoral radiography. In intraoral radiography, scatter radiation is reduced by using as small a beam as possible, open-ended PIDs, lead backing in the film package, and kVp settings of 65 and above.

Film contrast. Film contrast is determined by (1) the amount of radiation transmitted (object contrast), (2) the properties of the film, (3) intensifying screens, if used, (4) film processing, and (5) viewing conditions. Each of these factors is discussed in their respective sections. The important fact is that any secondary radiation or light that affects the film will decrease the desired contrast, or "fog" the film, which will degrade the image.

Image detail and definition

Image detail is the visual quality of a radiograph that depends on definition or sharpness. The factors that influence detail are (1) size of the tube focal or target area, (2) focal-film distance, (3) object-film distance, (4) movement of either patient or x-ray machine, (5) type of intensifying screen, if used, and (6) image contrast.

Size of tube focal (target) area. The smaller the focal area at the anode (see Fig. 1-15) of the x-ray, the better the image detail will be. As discussed in Chapter 1, the heat produced limits how small the focal area can be. The focal area in the tube is tilted, usually at an angle of 20 degrees to the cathode (Fig. 2-3), and when viewed from below the focal area appears to be smaller than it actually is. This is called the effective focal area, as contrasted to the actual focal area. The effective area is always smaller than the actual focal area. Most dental x-ray machines are equipped with the smallest focal area possible given the heat production restrictions.

Focal-film distance (FFD) and object-film distance (OFD). The ideal radiograph of an object, such as a tooth, in regard to definition, image enlargement, and distortion, can be made by meeting the following criteria:
1. Have a maximum focal-film distance. FFD is the distance between the focal spot (target) at the anode and the film in the patient's mouth. The maximum distance will enable the more parallel rays from the middle of the x-ray beam to strike the object, and not the more divergent x-rays from the periphery of the beam, which would cause image enlargement on the film (Fig. 2-4).
2. Have a minimum object-film distance. The tooth and the film should be as

Fig. 2-3. Diagram of the effective focal area and the actual focal area of an x-ray tube.

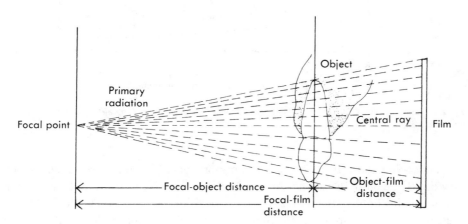

Fig. 2-4. Relationship between focal point, object, and film.

close together as possible. The closer they are, the less the enlargement there will be of the image on the film (Fig. 2-4).

3. Have the object and the film parallel to each other in their long axes and the central ray perpendicular to both (paralleling versus bisecting).

These are the optimum requirements. In intraoral radiography, because of anatomic restraints, it is impossible to meet all of these requirements at the same time.

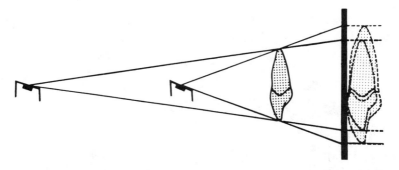

Fig. 2-5. Comparison of 8- and 16-inch focal-film distance. (Courtesy Rinn Corp., Elgin, Ill.)

Fig. 2-6. Relationship of image magnification to object-film distance and focal-film distance. (Courtesy Rinn Corp., Elgin, Ill.)

Focal-film distance. The most common focal-film distances used in dentistry are 8, 12, and 16 inches. An FFD of less than 8 inches may cause magnification of the image that is larger than the film (Fig. 2-5). As the FFD is increased to 12 or 16 inches, the magnification of the image decreases because the image is being formed by the more parallel x-rays from the center of the beam. However, this decrease in magnification is not a linear relationship beyond 16 inches. Fig. 2-6 shows that as the FFD is increased beyond 16 inches the percentage of magnification does not decrease significantly. Therefore using a 24-inch FFD does not give a significantly better image clinically than a 16-inch FFD, and there is no advantage in using this long FFD. The 16-inch FFD is the distance of choice. The extended or 16-inch focal-film distance also results in less tissue volume being exposed (see Chapter 4). The 16-inch FFD produces a better image and less radiation to the patient. For these reasons its use is strongly recommended.[1]

Fig. 2-7. Long beam tube head *(top)* and conventional tube head *(bottom)*. Note different position of x-ray tube itself that allows for increased focal-film distance.

Tube position. The x-ray tube is positioned in the anterior part of the head of the machine close to the PID or "cone" (Fig. 2-7). The rest of the head of the x-ray machine contains electric circuitry and cooling devices. The open-ended rectangle or cylinder, placed on the head of the machine, serves as the aiming device for the x-ray beam, and the length of this PID determines the focal distance to be used.

There was objection to the long cones as being bulky, cumbersome, and difficult to operate in small operatories. It also was said that the long cone tended to unbalance the head of the x-ray machine. With the increasing popularity of the paralleling technique and the need for an extended focal-film distance, a new design for the tube head was introduced. Fig. 2-7 illustrates the operation of the new design. The x-ray tube is placed in the rear part of the head of the machine, and the rest of the components are placed on both sides of the beam. The advantage of the design is found in the extended focal distance and the elimination of the long, bulky cone. The terms short cone and long cone are no longer appropriate. Cones are now outdated because of radiation hygiene, having been replaced by open-ended, lead-lined cylinders and rectangles, and also because the machine with the short cone may really have a long focal-film distance, depending on the placement of the x-ray tube in the head of the machine.

Inverse square law (Fig. 2-8). One of the factors that must be considered when choosing or changing an FFD is the inverse square law. It states that "the intensity of radiation varies inversely with the square of the distance." More simply stated, if the FFD is doubled, the exposure time is quadrupled. This assumes that the mA and kVp will remain the same.

Anode

Collimating device

Fig. 2-8. Inverse square law. The effect of distance on the intensity of the radiation.

As seen in Fig. 2-8, the intensity of the radiation at 16 inches is much less than it is at 8 inches, since it is spread out over 16 boxes. To achieve the same intensity of radiation, the exposure time must be increased by a factor of 4. In Fig. 2-8, the field size at 16 inches would be kept to 4 boxes by decreasing the aperture of the collimating device.

Before the advent of more sensitive films, the inverse square law presented more of a limiting factor than it does today. For instance, if one were using an 8-inch FFD at 1-second exposure and then changed to a 16-inch FFD, a 4-second exposure time would be necessary to produce a comparable film at the same mA and kVp. This 4-second exposure time would be inordinately long, and there could be patient movement. With the use of faster x-ray film and exposure times in the range of 2/10-second at an 8-inch FFD, a 16-inch FFD would need only 8/10-second exposure time. Clinically, 8/10-second exposure time, when compared with 2/10-second exposure time, presents no more or less problem with the patient movement. The same amount of radiation is reaching the film in the 8- and 16-inch techniques; it just takes greater time to achieve required x-ray intensity with the increased distance.

Another clinical application of the inverse square law is the positioning of

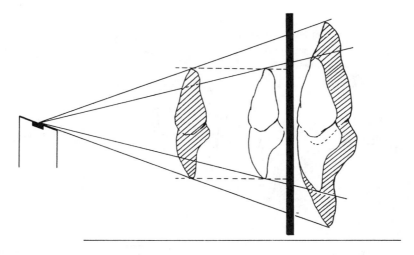

Fig. 2-9. Comparison of object-film distances and the effect on image magnification.

the PID almost touching the patient's face when taking intraoral radiographs. This will give the desired FFD, depending on the length of the PID. If the operator is careless in placement and does not approximate the skin, this will produce an increased FFD and decreased intensity of the x-ray beam by a factor of the square of the distance from the patient's face. A small distance, when squared, can lead to an underexposed film. Most dental offices will select an FFD and keep this technique constant.

Object-film distance. The closer the object (tooth, bone, etc.) is to the film, the better the detail and the enlargement will be (Fig. 2-9). The object-film distance will depend on the anatomy of the area of the mouth being radiographed and whether the paralleling or bisecting technique is used.

Image distortion and enlargement

Because of the anatomy of the mouth it is impossible to satisfy ideal criteria 2 and 3 (p. 32), which refer to object-film distance and parallelism between the object and the film. If the film is held close to the teeth, then the parallelism will be lost; if the teeth and film are to be parallel, there must be increased OFD.

This is the basis for the two techniques used in film placement for intraoral radiography: the paralleling technique and the bisecting-angle technique. The details of performing both these techniques, as well as their advantages and disadvantages, will be described in Chapters 7 and 8.

In the paralleling technique the film is held parallel to the long axis of the tooth. This results in an increased OFD in most areas of the mouth; that is, for the film to remain parallel to the tooth it must be positioned away from the tooth

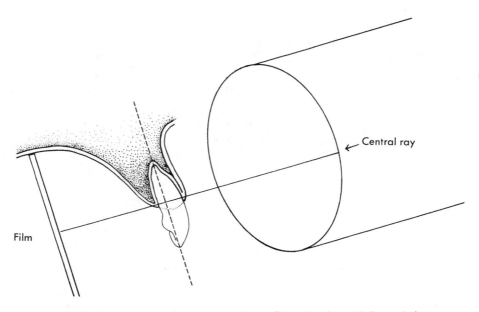

Fig. 2-10. Relationship of central ray, tooth, and film packet in paralleling technique.

(Fig. 2-10). The enlargement caused by the increased OFD is compensated for by using an increased FFD (12 or 16 inches). The use of the increased FFD is the reason for the misnomer "long cone technique." It is not the long cone that is of primary importance but the parallelism between the tooth and the film.

In the bisecting-angle technique the film is held as close to the tooth as possible. At this point the long axis of the tooth and the plane of the film cannot be parallel. A geometric trick is then used to project the proper image of the tooth onto the film. An imaginary line is drawn that bisects the angle formed by the long axis of the tooth and the plane of the dental film (Fig. 2-11). The central ray of the x-ray beam is then directed perpendicularly at this bisecting line. This will project the proper linear dimensions of the tooth onto the film without elongation or foreshortening.

Movement. There are two types of movement that will affect image detail—patient movement and x-ray source movement. Patient movement is controlled by good chairside technique and is discussed in later sections of this book. Source movement or tube and arm movement is caused by improper upkeep of x-ray equipment. If the arm or head moves or vibrates, image quality is compromised. There is no excuse for this type of error, and an effective quality control program should detect this malfunction. In many jurisdictions tube or arm movement is a violation of the Radiation Health Code.[2]

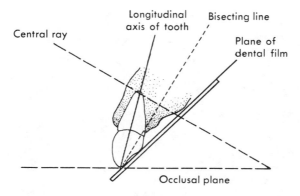

Central ray

Longitudinal
axis of tooth

Bisecting line

Plane of
dental film

Occlusal plane

Fig. 2-11. Relationship of central ray, tooth, and film packet in bisecting-angle technique.

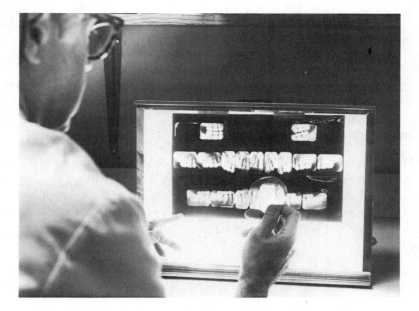

Fig. 2-12. Dentist viewing radiographs on an illuminating box.

Intensifying screens (film screen combinations). The use of intensifying screens and their effect on image definition are discussed in Chapter 9.

Viewing conditions (Fig. 2-12). Radiographs should always be looked at on an illuminator (view box). A magnifying glass can be used to look at fine changes. Ideally the room should be darkened when viewing radiographs. Radiographs should never be viewed by holding them up to the light on the unit or to the light from the window. Valuable information can be lost or never seen if the proper viewing conditions are not used and maintained.

Fig. 2-13. Intraoral film packet sizes, child (#0); narrow anterior (#1); adult size (#2); preformed bite-wing (#3); and occlusal (#4).

IMAGE RECEPTORS

The image receptors used in dentistry today are film, film screen combinations, xeroradiographic plates and the radiation detectors used in computed tomography. All of these use x-rays to generate an image on a receptor. In medicine, imaging systems are used that use x-rays, such as fluoroscopy, as are systems that do not use x-rays, such as ultrasound and magnetic resonance imaging (MRI).

Film

Film is by far still the most commonly used imaging system in dentistry. Intraoral packets come in three basic sizes (Fig. 2-13): child size, #0; adult size, #2; and narrow anterior film, #1. There are also occlusal film packets, #4, and preformed long bite-wing films, #3, available.

All the film packets must be light-tight and resistant to saliva seepage. These packets must have some degree of flexibility and should be easy to open in the darkroom.

The dental x-ray film packet has an outer plasticlike wrapper. Inside the wrapper is found the x-ray film, covered by black paper, and a lead-foil backing. The lead backing is placed on the side of the film away from the x-ray tube to absorb any unused radiation and prevent back-scattering secondary radiation from fogging the film (Fig. 2-14).

Waterproof outer package
Black paper
Film
Black paper
Lead foil backing
Waterproof outer covering

A

B

Fig. 2-14. A, Back of an opened dental film packet; **B,** Diagram of A.

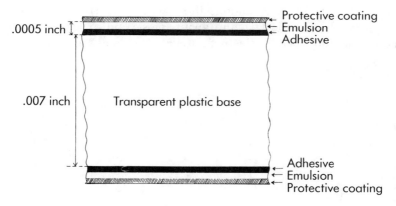

.0005 inch

Protective coating
Emulsion
Adhesive

.007 inch

Transparent plastic base

Adhesive
Emulsion
Protective coating

Fig. 2-15. Cross section diagram of film base and emulsion.

A film packet may contain one or two pieces of film. The so-called double film packet requires slightly more exposure time than the single film packet.

X-ray film is composed of a clear cellulose acetate film base coated with a emulsion of silver halide (usually silver bromide) grains suspended in a layer of gelatin (Fig. 2-15). It is the emulsion that is sensitive to x-rays, visible light, and static electricity. The film base is coated on both sides and thus is called a double emulsion. This allows less radiation to be used than when there was only an emulsion on one side of the film. Clinically, this means that a radiograph can be correctly viewed from either side. Previously, with single-emulsion film, the film had to be viewed from the side with the emulsion on it. The film also has a button or dot on it. This is a small convex-concave area that helps one to orient the developed film in mounting (see Chapter 12).

Film sensitivity. The size of the silver bromide crystals, the thickness of the emulsion, and the presence of special radiosensitive dyes determines the film speed, or film sensitivity. Film sensitivity determines how much radiation for what period of time (mAs) will be necessary to produce an image on the film.

Films that are more sensitive require less mAs and are said to have greater film speed; these are the fast films. Films that require more mAs are less sensitive to radiation and are called slower films. The size of the silver bromide crystals is the main factor in determining the film speed: the larger the crystals, the faster the film.

Film sensitivity is compared or expressed by means of a characteristic or H & D (Hurter and Driffield) curve (Fig. 2-16). The curve gives the relationship between radiation exposure to the film and the resulting film density. A fast film would require less exposure to produce a desired density than a slower film.

Different film manufacturers will give different brand names to their various film speed types. There is no slow-speed film being made today. At 65 kVp and 10 mA, slow film would need an average exposure time of about 3 seconds per film. Under the same conditions the intermediate-speed film would need about 1½ seconds and the fast film about ³⁄₁₀-second exposure per film. One manufacturer's "ultraspeed" (Eastman Kodak Co.) may be equal to another's

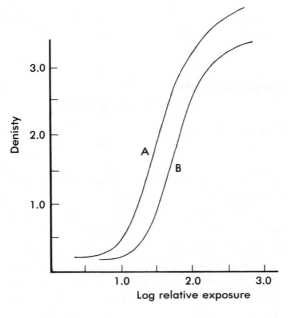

Fig. 2-16. H & D curve. Note that film A requires less exposure to achieve a given film density than film B.

"lightning" or "very fast" film speed. It is obvious that some standards and nomenclature are necessary. Film speed is designated into groups by the American National Standards Institute (ANSI) using the letters A through F, A being the slowest film and F the fastest. To get comparable film sensitivities when changing from one manufacturer to another, one should consult the ANSI speed group ratings found on the package and not be misled by descriptive names.

Presently, there are only two film speed groups that should be used, groups E and D. The American Dental Association (ADA) and the American Academy of Oral and Maxillofacial Radiology currently recommend that E speed film should be used.[1,2] The ADA further recommends that films in a speed group slower than group D should not be used.[1] Certain health codes forbid the use of film slower than group D.[3] Group E speed film is twice as fast as group D film, and thus the patient receives half the radiation exposure for a comparable diagnostic film.[4]

Film definition and detail. The definition or detail on a film is also dependent on the size of the silver bromide crystals. The larger crystals, theoretically, although they allow for reduced exposure time, give poorer definition when compared with the smaller, slower crystals.

The dilemma is whether to reduce the amount of radiation the patient receives by using fast films with large crystals, thereby sacrificing definition, or to increase exposure time by using small crystals to give better definition and thereby increase radiation exposure. This is largely a theoretical dilemma, because the human eye, which must view the finished radiograph, cannot easily distinguish between the definition on group E speed films and that on group D films. The debate today is on the image quality of D versus E film. The literature strongly suggests that it is difficult to tell the difference between films and that the decrease in radiation far outweighs the slight possible loss of definition.[5]

Film fog. An x-ray film is fogged when the whole or part of the radiograph is darkened by sources other than the radiation of the primary beam to which the film was exposed. Fogging degrades the diagnostic image. The following are several sources of fogging:

1. Chemical fog results from an imbalance or exhaustion of processing solutions (see Chapter 6).
2. Light fog results from unintentional exposure of light to which the film emulsion is sensitive, either before or during processing (see Chapter 6).
3. Scattered radiation fog results from radiation striking the film from sources other than the intentional exposure of the primary beam. Examples of this would be scatter from the patient or unprotected storage of films before or after exposure.

REFERENCES

1. American Dental Association, Council on Dental Materials, Instruments, and Equipment: Recommendations in radiographic practices: an update, 1988, J Am Dent Assoc 118:115-117, 1988.
2. American Academy of Oral and Maxillofacial Radiology: Position paper on rectangular collimation and E speed film Oral Surg Oral Med Oral Path (in press).
3. New York City Health Code, Article 175, Feb 1981.
4. Silha RE: Methods for reducing patient exposure combined with Kodak Ekta speed dental x-ray film, Dent Radiogr Photogr 54:4, 1981.
5. Kantor ML, Reiskin AB, and Lurie AG: A clinical comparison of x-ray film for detection of proximal surface caries, J Am Dent Assoc 111:967-969, 1985.

3

Biologic effects of radiation

Much has been written, not only in scientific journals but also in the media, about the effects of ionizing radiation, both manmade and naturally occurring, on human beings and the environment. This growing concern about the biologic effects of ionizing radiation is not limited to the scientific community but is evident in the public sector and at all levels of government. On television our patients view demonstrations against nuclear power plants and nuclear weapons, they read about radon gas in homes, and there are discussions of arms treaties to keep radiation out of the atmosphere. Events such as the near-fatal nuclear accident at Three Mile Island, Pennsylvania, and the catastrophe at Chernobyl in the USSR have heightened public awareness to the dangers of low-level radiation. Fear and uncertainty aroused by these events may lead some patients to refuse necessary diagnostic radiographic examinations or even avoid dental visits completely. Health professionals need to be informed about risks and benefits of dental radiation so that they may anticipate and allay unfounded fears.

Information about ionizing radiation that reaches the public from the media can be misleading and confusing. The latest data indicate that radiation from medicine and dentistry, including nuclear medicine, accounts for about 15% of the average annual dose equivalent to the US population.[1] This, however, is the largest source of manmade radiation to which the population is exposed. At the same time as one talks about the risk of exposure one should consider the diagnostic benefits and health-preserving or lifesaving consequences of the radiation.

Patient reaction can vary from questioning the need for dental radiographs to outright refusal. The dental auxiliary must face this patient reaction and, with the support of the dentist, be able to explain to the patient the biologic effects of dental x-ray exposure and the diagnostic benefits that will be derived.

Ionizing radiation does produce biologic changes in living tissue, and patients should not be misled into believing that dental x-rays have no effect on human cells. The old reply to patient queries regarding radiation safety that claimed that "dental x-rays are safe because the dosage is so small it doesn't matter" will no longer satisfy informed health care consumers.

The question is no longer whether there is a risk from x-rays, but how much of a risk there is. In determining whether radiographs should be used, the dentist must weigh the potential harm of dental x-rays against the benefit the diagnostic information will yield. In dental radiography performed under optimum conditions and when indicated, the diagnostic benefits far outweigh the potential risks.

Our objective for the patient is to use the least possible amount of radiation to obtain the greatest diagnostic yield. For the dental auxiliary, as well as the dentist, the objective is to achieve occupational radiation exposure as close to zero as possible. To achieve these objectives, the dental auxiliary must fully understand the subjects of radiation biology and protection. Explanations to patients will then be meaningful, and the assistant or hygienist will feel at ease working in an environment where diagnostic radiation is used.

EFFECTS OF IONIZING RADIATION

When a dental radiograph is taken, not all the x-rays reach the film and some even penetrate beyond it. Some of the x-ray energy of the primary beam is absorbed by the skin, bones, teeth, and other body tissues that lie in its path. Tissues that do not lie in the path of the primary beam absorb the energy of the secondary radiation that comes from the patient as a result of the interaction of the primary beam. It is the differential absorption of the x-ray photons by the hard tissues, teeth, and bones that enables us to distinguish various structures on the finished radiograph. What is the effect of this x-ray energy absorption on the various tissues, and how is it manifested?

The human body, like all living organisms, functions through the existence of ions in its organs, tissues, and cells. These ions are electrically charged particles that originate in the water, salts, proteins, carbohydrates, and fats that are the principal components of our bodies. The ions affect the many complex functions that maintain the health of the body and return it to health after illness. Ions are ever present in a finely balanced state, or equilibrium, so that precise control over the reactions concerned with body function can be maintained. If an overabundance of ions occurs, the surplus must be removed immediately if health is to be maintained; illness will also occur if an insufficient number of necessary ions is available for essential functioning. Special ions maintain the proper body environment for such things as respiration, muscular activity, speech, and digestion. X-ray exposure, depending on the amount, can upset this delicately balanced state because of the x-rays' ability to cause ionization.

The mechanism of this ionization or the ability to produce ions was described in Chapter 1. In the case of interaction with or penetration of the human body, extra ions become available. These extra ions can upset the fine ionic balance that exists. If the amount of radiation exposure is large, there will be a great ionic upset, and the body will react by showing signs of injury or illness. It is important to understand that x-rays are ionizing radiation and, as such, have the potential to affect the health of the human body.

UNITS OF RADIATION MEASUREMENT

Before we can talk logically about the potential effects of dental radiation, we must have some means of measuring the radiation quantitatively. The settings on the control panel of the dental x-ray machine are not measurements of the x-ray energy (ionizing radiation) produced; the kilovoltage and milliamperage are indications of the quality and quantity of the electric energy put into the x-ray machine, and the timer provides a reading of how long the ionizing radiation will be produced. The HVL, although a measurement of the x-ray beam, describes the penetration and the quality of the beam. The units of measure that commonly have been employed, each with its own application, have been the roentgen, the *rad* (for radiation absorbed dose), and the rem (roentgen equivalent man). To standardize units to the metric system, these conventional units are being replaced by those of the Systeme Internationale (SI). The new units are the coulomb per kilogram (c/kg), the gray (Gy), and the sievert (Sv). This text will use the conventional units with the SI units in parentheses.

Exposure

The unit most commonly used to measure the amount of energy, or ionizing radiation, being produced by the x-ray machine is called the *roentgen* and is abbreviated as R. The milliroentgen is $1/1000$ of a roentgen; because the exposures in dental radiology are small, they are often expressed in milliroentgens, or mR (1000 mR = 1 R). The SI unit for exposure would be coulomb/kilogram (c/kg), l c/kg = $3.88 \times 10 - 3$ R.

The roentgen is a measurement of ionization in air. It is defined as the quantity of radiation that produces one electrostatic charge in 1 cc of air. The roentgen is our measuring standard for radiation. just as we have to know what an inch is before we can compare lengths, we have a standard—the roentgen—to measure radiation. Just as there are rulers and scales, there are ionization chambers that are calibrated in roentgens. An ionization chamber placed in front of a dental x-ray machine PID can indicate how many roentgens are being produced per second (Fig. 3-1). This is called the exposure rate or output of the machine. Since it is a measurement of ionization in air, it is measured in roentgens per second. A well-calibrated dental x-ray machine will have an output in the range of 0.7 to 1 R per second. If a patient had a radiograph taken with such a machine and the exposure time was 1 second, the facial exposure of the patient would be 0.7 R (0.7 R/sec $\times$ 1 sec = 0.7 R).

Dose

The critical factor in discussing the effects of radiation is not the amount of radiation at a point in air, but rather the amount of energy absorbed by tissue at a specific point. To express the amount of energy absorbed by a tissue, we

Fig. 3-1. Ionization chamber measuring the output of dental x-ray machine.

use the rad or the gray. The rad is a unit of absorbed dose (radiation absorbed dose) and is defined as 100 ergs of energy per gram of absorber (tissue). The millirad is $\frac{1}{1000}$ of a rad. The unit for the absorbed dose in SI units is the gray (1 rad = 0.01 Gy or 1 Gy = 100 rads).

Dose equivalent

Different types of radiation on a rad-for-rad basis will have different effects on living tissue. Neutrons for example will have a greater effect on tissue than will x or gamma radiation. The term *dose equivalent* is defined as the dose multiplied by the quality factor Q and is expressed in units of rem. The millirem is 1/1000 of a rem. The unit for the dose equivalent in SI units is the sievert (1 rem = 0.01 Sv or 1 Sv = 100 rems). The quality factor by definition for x-radiation and gamma radiation is one *1* so that the dose equivalent in rems (sieverts) is equal to the dose in rads (grays).

In terms of the effects of dental radiation, the rad (gray) and the rem (sievert) are identical and the roentgen is approximately equal to both (roentgen = rad = rem).

RADIATION UNITS

Conventional Unit	Definition	SI Unit	Definition	Conversion
roentgen (R)	1 esu/cc of air	coulomb/kg		1 c/kg = 3876 R
rad	100 erg/g	gray (Gy)	1 j/kg	1 G = 100 rad
rem	rad × Q	sievert (Sv)	Gy × Q	1 SV = 100 rem

BASIC CONCEPTS

Exposure and dose

Although the terms are often interchanged, there is a very definite distinction between radiation *exposure* and *dose*. Exposure is the measure of ionization in the air produced by x-ray or gamma radiation; it is the quantity of radiation in an area to which the patient is exposed. The radiation dose is the amount of energy absorbed per unit mass of tissue at a particular site. In dentistry, the patient is exposed to a certain amount of radiation, some of which is absorbed by tissue in different parts of the body; this is the dose to the area. Exposure should be expressed in roentgens (coulombs/kg), and dose should be expressed in rads (grays) or rems (sieverts).

Localized radiation and total body exposure (Fig. 3-2)

It is important to differentiate between localized radiation and the total body exposure. When a dental radiograph is taken, the patient's face is exposed to an x-ray beam that is 2¾ inches in diameter (with circular collimation). This is a localized exposure to that area of the body. A rad of radiation to the localized area means that each gram of body tissue in that area absorbs 1 rad of radiation. A rad of total body radiation means that each gram of tissue in the entire body absorbs 1 rad of radiation. In dentistry, the machine delivers a localized exposure that results in a total body exposure much less than the facial exposure. In fact, the total body exposure from a dental radiograph is approximately ¹⁄₁₀,₀₀₀ of the facial exposure.

When discussions of dental x-ray dosages appear in magazine articles, or if patients quote such articles, it is important to determine whether localized exposure or total body exposure is being discussed. For instance, what is the facial exposure of radiation to the patient from a full-mouth survey of radiographs? An average *full-mouth survey* at 70 kVp, 10 mA, using ANSI group E film, will produce a skin exposure to the patient's face of approximately 2 to 3 R. This is not the total body exposure but a localized exposure. The total body dose could be approximated by dividing the localized dose, 3 R, by 10,000.

Fig. 3-2. A, Localized exposure; B, Total body exposure.

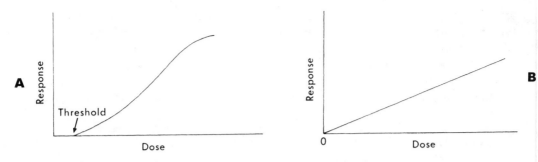

Fig. 3-3. Dose response curve. **A,** Threshold curve; **B,** Nonthreshold linear type.

The most common misuse of such data occurs when referring to the recommendation of the National Bureau of Standards that the total body dose for people working with ionizing radiation should not exceed 5 R in any 1 year. The misstatement then is, "You are allowed 5 R per year, and when your dentist x-rays your entire mouth he exposes you to 3 R of radiation." The mistake here is equating the total body dose to the localized dose in addition to using an occupational exposure for a patient exposure. The truer figure to compare the dental facial dose with the 5 R would be 0.0003 R.

Dose response curve

The dose response curve is an important concept because it illustrates the two possible biologic responses to a harmful agent such as ionizing radiation. Fig. 3-3, *A,* is a threshold curve indicating that below a certain level (the threshold) there is no response to the agent. If this concept is applied to dental radiation, there would be a level below which radiographs would be "perfectly safe" since there would be no biologic response below that level. This is not thought to be the case for ionizing radiation (Fig. 3-3, *B*). This curve indicates that any dose of radiation, regardless of how small, will produce some degree of biologic response. Therefore, dental x-rays do produce biologic changes in the tissues of the patients who receive them. It is important to realize that most of the data that produce such a dose response curve for humans come from studying the effects of large doses of radiation on populations such as atomic bomb survivors. In the low-dose range for humans, where dental x-rays fall, little has been documented. The line is therefore an extrapolation based on animal and cellular experiments. The consensus is that ionizing radiation is a linear, nonthreshold relationship.[2]

Somatic and genetic effects

All the cells in the body, with the exception of the reproductive cells (sperm and ova), are included in the grouping of somatic tissue. Changes in these cells are not passed on to succeeding generations of the species. For example, a cancerous skin condition will not be passed on to an offspring. Somatic tissue can be affected by radiation and some cells may die, be altered, or even recover, but none of these effects will be seen in the somatic tissue of the progeny.

Changes in genetic cells are passed on to succeeding generations and are referred to as genetic mutations. There are many other agents besides ionizing radiation that have been found to be mutanogenic, including a variety of chemicals, certain drugs, and even elevated body temperatures. Background radiation also accounts for a portion of naturally occurring mutations. Some of the mutations that have been manifested have been positive and have added to the so-called evolution of the species. A mutation may be recessive and carried in the progeny for many generations before becoming clinically evident.

With the increase in low-level, man-made radiation in recent years, the original concern dealt mainly with the possible genetic effects on succeeding generations. Recently the concern has turned toward somatic tissue, and cancer induction in the blood-forming organs in particular. Leukemia is now believed to be the major risk of chronic low-level radiation.

The National Academy of Sciences has recommended that "the average exposure of the populations' reproductive cells to radiation above natural background levels should be limited to 10 roentgens from conception to age 30."[3] There is some slight genetic risk from scattered radiation in dental radiography. The U.S. Public Health Service reported in 1969 before the introduction of group E film that the mean gonadal dose from all dental films is less than 0.1 millirad (0.0001 rad).[4] These values compare favorably with the average daily whole-body exposure of 0.3 mR from natural background radiation.[5]

Acute and chronic effects

The short-term (acute) effects of radiation result from high doses of whole body radiation, usually over 100 rads. The clinical effect of the exposure, which may vary from mild and transient illness to death, may occur minutes, hours, or weeks after the acute exposure. The median lethal dose for humans is estimated to be 450 rads. It is obvious that in dentistry, we are not concerned with acute radiation doses.

Long-term (chronic) effects of radiation may be seen years after the original exposures. There may be cumulative effects of acute and/or chronic exposures to the somatic cells over the patient's lifetime, as well as genetic effects on future generations.

Direct and indirect effects

The effects of ionizing radiation on tissue may be direct, as when the ionizing radiation alters or destroys cells that lie in the direct path of the radiation beam. The effects may also be indirect, as when the impaired function of the radiated tissue adversely influences other tissues in the body. An example of an indirect effect would be the production of a chemically changed hormone that could not properly regulate tissue elsewhere in the body.

Latent period and cell recovery

The latent period is the time that elapses between the exposure to ionizing radiation and the appearance of clinical symptoms. This time may vary from hours to years, depending on the magnitude of the exposure and the tissues involved. Not all radiation-induced changes in tissue cells are permanent. Depending on the time interval, the dose, and the sensitivity of the affected cells to radiation, the cells' repair processes may be sufficient to effect recovery from the radiation.

Dose rate

The *dose rate,* the rate at which exposure to ionizing radiation occurs and absorption takes place, is a very important factor in determining what the effects will be. Since there is cell recovery from radiation, a specific dose will produce less damage if it is fractionated over a period of time. In dentistry, the time interval between exposures, excluding retakes and working films, is usually months or years, further minimizing the effects.

Long-term effects

The long-term effects of radiation manifest themselves years after the exposure. The latent period is very long. These delayed effects may be from an acute exposure or a series of low-level exposures. A low-level exposure is considered to be under 5 rems (0.05 sieverts).

It is important to remember that there is no specific disease associated solely with the long-term effects of radiation. Cancer can be caused by radiation, but it is also caused by smoking, chronic irritants, and exposure to certain chemicals.

Since there is no specific radiation disease, the long-term effects of radiation express themselves in human populations as a statistical increase in the incidence of certain disease. One can study the incidence of diseases in irradiated populations and compare to nonirradiated groups. The atomic bomb survivors and the incidence of leukemias among them is a good example of this type of evaluation of the long-term effects. Evaluating the long-term effects of dental x-rays, where the dose is low, would require large populations over a long period, since the latent period for radiation-induced cancer—even from large doses—ranges from years to decades.[6]

Risk estimates

Since there is no effective way of analyzing the cause of a radiations induced cancer on a case-by-case basis, we must look to dosages in irradiated populations and the number of cancers in these populations. This number is then compared to nonirradiated populations and the difference is expressed as the risk factor.

Risk factors are expressed as the number of cases or deaths from a specific disease per million persons of population. Estimates have been made of the number of cases of cancer for all body organs induced per 1 million dental examinations. For a full-mouth survey taken with round collimation the estimate is 6 to 17 cases per million examinations. If rectangular collimation is used, the risk is estimated to be 1 or 2 cases per million examinations.[7]

These numbers may seem quite threatening, but they should be compared with risks that our patients take in everyday life. Activities that are rated at 1 in 1 million risks of fatal outcomes in everyday life include traveling 10 miles on a bicycle, 300 miles in an automobile, 1000 miles on an airline, or smoking 1.4 cigarettes a day.[8] It is obvious that we readily accept one in a million risks in everyday living, even though there may not be and in many cases obviously there is no health benefit.

TISSUE SENSITIVITY

There is a wide variation among tissues in their sensitivity to ionizing radiation and thus the amount of radiation required to produce damage. The same dose of radiation will have a different degree of effect on different types of cells in the same organism. Young, rapidly dividing, non-differentiated cells, such as those found in the abdomen of the pregnant dental patient, are more radiosensitive than older cells. In addition to the age of the cell and its rate of differentiation, tissues vary in their sensitivity to radiation. Grouping tissues and organs in descending order of sensitivity to radiation, we have the following[5]:

High sensitivity:	Lymphoid organs
	Bone marrow
	Testes
	Intestines
Intermediate:	Fine vasculature
	Growing cartilage
	Growing bone
Low:	Salivary glands
	Lungs
	Kidneys
	Liver
	Optic lens

Certain organs and tissues have been designated as "critical" because they are exposed to more radiation than others when dental radiographs are taken. The tissues and organs designated as critical are the skin, thyroid, eye, and hematopoietic and genetic tissue.

Background radiation

Background radiation is a form of ionizing radiation, both naturally occurring and manmade, present in the environment. This naturally occurring radiation has always been present on earth, but the manmade component has been increasing as a result of fallout from nuclear testing and radioactive wastes from industry. It would be helpful to know the level of background radiation and its sources, so that dental radiation exposure can be put in its proper perspective.

An estimate of the average personal exposure, weighted from different sources to approximate a "total body exposure," has been tabulated and is shown below.[1] This report shows an estimated average annual dose of 300 millirem (3 millisieverts) due to natural background sources. With the addition of the average contributions of medical and dental procedures the total annual average population exposure is about 360 millirems (3.6 millisieverts). Of the total exposure 55% is from exposure to radon.

AVERAGE ANNUAL EXPOSURE TO U.S. POPULATION

Source	Dose (millirems)
Natural Sources	
Radon	200
Cosmic radiation	27
Soil and building materials	28
Internal radioactivity	39
Occupational	0.9
Nuclear fuel cycle	0.5
Consumer products	9.0
Miscellaneous	0.06
Medical and dental	53

These data help to compare dental exposure with background exposure. From the data and from known outputs of dental x-ray machines it can be said that total body radiation from a four-film bite-wing examination using rectangular collimation and E-speed film is equivalent to about 12 hours of background. Using a round beam and D-speed film it can be as high as 82 hours of background.

Patient dosage

Ample evidence in the literature substantiates the adverse effects of radiation in high doses. The problem is that no direct evidence exists of such effects from dental diagnostic doses, but there is also no evidence that proves that there are no adverse effects. To treat a patient without current and diagnostic radiographs is doing a disservice to the patient and leaves the dentist unprotected against possible legal action. Radiographs are an integral part of modern dental practice. Our goal in dental radiography is to use the least amount of radiation to satisfy the patient's diagnostic needs, that is, minimize the exposure while maximizing the diagnostic yield. In our efforts to minimize the amount of radiation, we must also be guided by the *ALARA principle*, which means "as low as reasonably achievable." The radiation exposure to our patients should be reduced as much as possible within the dental office without excessive cost or inconvenience to the patient.

How do we evaluate these effects of ionizing radiation and the weight of the dental component? There is no specific disease that can be attributed solely to the long-term effects of ionizing radiation. As previously mentioned, leukemia is not caused by x-ray exposure alone but is probably the result of the interaction of several factors. Animal experimentation has been done, but direct extrapolation of the results of human populations is not always reliable. Data gained from acute exposures of humans, such as the victims of Hiroshima or industrial accidents, that are then extrapolated downward to low doses also have their limitations. Furthermore, the incidence of the diseases we are concerned with is low, so to relate an increased incidence with population exposure to ionizing radiations, it is necessary to study large populations.

Dental auxiliaries and dentists, because of their involvement with low-level ionizing radiation, should be aware of the consequences of chronic exposure for their patients. In this manner they are better equipped to make the essential risk-versus-benefit decision before making x-ray exposures.

The following examples of specific tissue exposures from dental x-ray exposure and the critical levels of these tissues enable us to say that the benefits derived from dental x-ray exposure, when used judiciously under proper conditions, far outweigh any possible risk.

Skin. Erythema (reddening of the skin) is the usual effect of radiation and is not a major risk in dental radiography. Its importance lies in that the skin dose is the most commonly reported value for dental x-ray examinations. The skin dose has limitations in that (1) it is easily penetrated and does not reflect a dose to deeper tissues, (2) it varies greatly with the kVp used, and (3) it is less sensitive than many other tissues exposed during dental radiography.

The threshold erythema dose (TED), the amount of radiation needed to produce an erythema or reddening of the most sensitive individual, is 250 R in a 14-day period.[9] Assuming an exposure rate of 0.7 R per second from a dental x-ray machine, using ANSI group E film, more than 500 dental exposures in a 14-day period would be necessary to produce an erythema in the most sensitive patient. Clinically, this is an absurd possibility, and it is not surprising then that there are no reported cases of erythema as a result of exposure to dental radiographs.

Eyes. Exposure to ionizing radiation in high doses to the lens of the eye can induce cataract formation. The required dose to produce this change has been reported in the range of 200 to 500 rads (2 to 5 Gy),[10] while the mean corneal surface dose for a full-mouth series has been reported to be about 0.188 rad (18.8 Gy).[11] The lens of the eye is exposed to radiation during intraoral radiography, but the risk of cataract formation is extremely low.

Thyroid. The thyroid gland, which is particularly radiosensitive, may lie in the beam of primary radiation in some dental views. Malignant changes have been reported in the thyroid glands in a group of patients who received x-ray therapy for tinea capitis (ringworm of the scalp).[12] The dose to the thyroid in these patients was estimated to be 6 rads. Presently, the thyroid exposure for a full-mouth series is about 47 mR (0.47 mGy),[5] or about 0.15% of the exposure in the tinea capitis studies. The dose to this radiosensitive tissue should be kept to an absolute minimum, especially in children. This can be accomplished by the use of a lead thyroid collar and the paralleling technique.

Bone marrow. It is now thought that the greatest somatic hazard to patients from dental x-rays is leukemia induction.[13] The red bone marrow is one of the blood-forming organs of the body. The significant hematopoietic bone marrow exposed to dental x-rays is located in the mandible, the calvarium of the skull, and the cervical spine. The calvarium and cervical spine are exposed to primary radiation in extraoral and panoramic radiography. The bone marrow of the mandible is the major dental concern, and it represents only 1.2% of all body active bone marrow.

White and Rose[14] published a report that will help the auxiliary and the dentist discuss the risk of leukemia with patients. They compared the higher background radiation in Denver, Colorado, due to high elevation and thus increased cosmic ray exposure, to bone marrow exposure from dental examinations. The report states, "If a person in an average location in the United States were to receive a full-mouth intraoral periapical and panoramic examination every 4 months for the rest of his life, he would incur only the same risk, in terms of bone marrow exposure, as a person living in Denver who was not exposed to dental radiography."

The leukemia risk, then, is very low but still exists. However, with judicious use of radiation and proper technique, the diagnostic benefit derived outweighs the slight risk.

It has been demonstrated for some time that there are no changes seen in the complete blood count (CBC) after dental x-ray examination.[15] This refutes an outdated report, still often cited in the lay press, that claimed significant blood changes after dental x-rays.[16]

Pregnancy. As previously mentioned, the nondifferentiated, rapidly dividing fetal cells are extremely radiosensitive; hence the concern for pregnant patients.

A panel of dental radiologists recently considered the appropriateness of dental radiographs for pregnant patients.[17] They concluded that the guidelines for taking radiographs for patients (discussed in Chapter 4) need not be altered for the pregnant patient. They pointed out that the concept of avoiding radiography during pregnancy generally applies to procedures in which the fetus or embryo would be in or near the primary x-ray beam. In dentistry the primary beam is limited to the head and neck region, and the only radiation the fetus would be exposed to would be secondary radiation. Uterine doses for a full-mouth series without using a lead apron have been shown to be less than 1 millirem.[18] As we have seen, the uterine dose from naturally occurring background during the 9 months of pregnancy can be expected to be about 225 mrem (2.25 mSv) based on the background doses of 300 mrem (3 mSv) per year. With these factors there seems to be no scientific reason to preclude an indicated dental x-ray examination during pregnancy. Radiographs in some cases may have to be deferred during pregnancy for purely psychological reasons.

As we will see in Chapter 4 (p. 73), there is no occupational hazard for the pregnant dentist or auxiliary, because when appropriate precautionary procedures are followed, the occupational dose will be zero.

Gonads (sperm cells and ova). The reproductive cells (sperm and ova) are very radiosensitive. Sterilization from an acute exposure from the dental x-ray beam is an impossibility; 400 R is needed in the male and 625 R in the female to cause sterility.

REFERENCES

1. National Council on Radiation Protection and Measurements: Ionizing radiation exposure of the population of the United States, Report No 93, 1987, Washington, DC, The Council.
2. National Academy of Sciences–National Research Council: The effects on populations of exposure to low levels of ionizing radiation, BEIR V. Washington, DC, 1990, National Academy Press.
3. National Academy of Sciences–National Research Council: The biological effects of atomic radiation, Washington, DC, 1952.
4. Population dose from x-rays: US 1964 HEW Publication #2001, Washington, DC, 1969.
5. Goaz PW and White SC: Oral radiology, St Louis, 1987, The CV Mosby Co.
6. Bebbe GW, Kato H and Land CE: Studies of the mortality of A-bomb survivors 1950-1974, Radiat Res 73:138-201, July 1978.
7. Danforth RA and Gibbs SJ: Diagnostic dental radiation, what is the risk? J Calif Dent Assoc 8:28-35, 1980.
8. Wilson R: Risks caused by low levels of pollution, Yale J Biol Med 51:37-51, 1978.
9. Richard AG: How hazardous is dental radiography? Oral Surg 14:1, Jan 1961.
10. International Commission on Radiological Protection, Radiosensitivity, and Patient Distribution of Dose: Publication 14, Oxford, 1969, Pergamon Press.
11. Greer DF: Determination and analysis of absorbed dose resulting from various intraoral radiographic techniques, Oral Surg 34:1, July 1972.
12. Pentel L: Current perspectives on radiation, NYJ Dent 45:3, March 1975.
13. White SC and Frey NW: An estimation of somatic hazards to the US population from dental radiography, Oral Surg 43:1, January 1977.
14. White SC and Rose TC: Absorbed bone marrow dose in certain dental radiographic techniques, J Am Dent Assoc 98:553-558, 1979.
15. Budowsky J et al: Lack of effect of exposure to radiation during intraoral roentgenographic examinations as post examination blood studies, J Am Dent Assoc 55:199, Aug 1957.
16. Nolan WE: Radiation hazards to the patient from oral roentgenography, J Am Dent Assoc 47:681, Dec 1953.
17. US Department of Health and Human Services, Public Health Service, FDA: The selection of patients for x-ray examinations, dental radiographic examinations, HSS/PHS/FDA 88-8273:10-21, 1987
18. Gibbs SJ et al: Radiation doses to sensitive organs from intraoral dental radiography, Dentomax Radiol 17:15-23, 1987.

4

Radiation protection

We will discuss the problem of radiation protection from the perspective of the two major concerns: the patient and the operator. Of the two we will see that the concern for the operator is the easier to deal with, because there are exact limits that can be easily adhered to.

PATIENT PROTECTION

In patient protection, the objective is to use the least amount of radiation to achieve the maximum diagnostic results. The patient must be protected from excessive or unnecessary primary radiation and the resulting secondary radiation. Through the use of safe, well-calibrated x-ray machines, rectangular collimation, film-holding devices, E-speed film, lead aprons, rare earth intensifying screens and thyroid collars, proper shielding, good chairside and darkroom techniques, and sound professional judgment in selection criteria, this goal can be met.

Primary radiation is the energy contained by the x-rays that come from the target of the x-ray tube. The primary radiation is collimated by the lead diaphragm and filtered of its softer less penetrating wavelengths by aluminum filters. It is then referred to as the *useful beam*. All other radiation can be considered secondary radiation. *Secondary radiation* is defined as radiation that comes from any matter being struck by primary radiation. The scattered radiation that results from the interaction of the useful beam and the patient's face is a form of secondary radiation (Fig. 4-1). Secondary radiation, besides being harmful to both patient and operator, will degrade the diagnostic image of the film, because the scattered rays will produce film fog on the radiograph.

EQUIPMENT

All dental x-ray machines manufactured after 1974 must meet federal diagnostic equipment performance standards.[1] There were no federal standards for x- ray machines manufactured or installed before 1974. It is important to remember that the federal standards do not regulate diagnostic equipment users such as dentists, but only the equipment itself. However, most state or local gov-

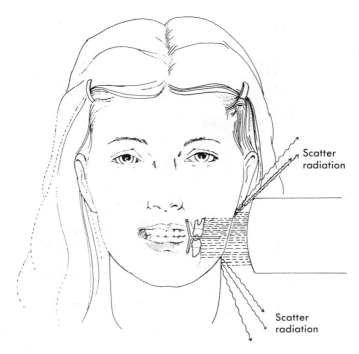

Scatter radiation

Scatter radiation

Fig. 4-1. Production of scatter radiation of primary beam by interaction with patient's face.

ernments also regulate equipment and have radiation health codes that pertain to the use of radiation. So the federal government regulates the manufacture and installation of x-ray machines and state and local governments regulate how they are used. Depending on the local radiation code, dental offices, clinics, and dental schools will be inspected every 1 to 3 years to monitor equipment performance and the barriers and procedures used when taking radiographs. Usually a fee is charged for this inspection, and many jurisdictions also require a fee for licensure to use x-ray machines.

Tube head and arm

Head leakage. The term head leakage refers to radiation that escapes through the protective shielding of the x-ray tube head. The only radiation that should leave the tube head is the primary beam. Radiation leakage exposes the patient unnecessarily and should not occur in a properly functioning x-ray unit. Leakage is a violation of the federal performance standards and local radiation codes.[1] This is not a common problem, because x-ray units are well built, if the unit is not abused in use or moving, head leakage is unlikely to occur.

Drift. The tube head of the dental x-ray machine should not evidence any drift in any direction after positioning for an exposure (see Fig. 1-1). The move-

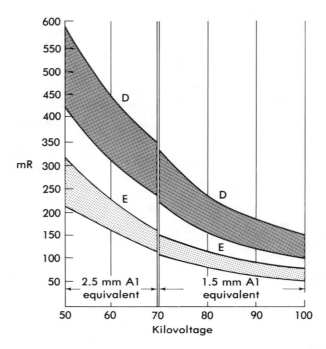

Fig. 4-2. Acceptable x-ray exposure ranges speed group D and E films. Note the increased exposure in the low kVp range and that the exposure with speed group E is about one-half that of speed group D. (Courtesy: Department of Health and Human Services.)

ment can cause a blurred image or position the central ray off the film, resulting in a "cone cut." If the tube head drifts, the arm should be repaired immediately. The patient or the auxillary should never hold the tube head in place during an exposure. Checking for tube head drift in all directions is an important step in an office quality assurance program.

Kilovoltage and milliamperage seconds. These technique factors control proper penetration and film density and contrast. As explained in Chapter 2, the mAs' contribution to the patient's radiation exposure is determined by the film speed and the FFD. The choice of kVp, however, will affect the contrast of the film and the radiation dose. The patient's skin exposure decreases as the kVp increases, but the dose to deeper tissues and the amount of scatter radiation increases. At present, there is some debate about the best kVp within the 65 to 90 range that should be used in dentistry.[2] A kilovoltage that is best suited for the diagnostic needs should be used. There is no question that kVp below 65 should not be used, because the exposure to the patient per film is nearly doubled when using a kVp below the acceptable range (Fig. 4-2).

Filtration. Because of the enactment of the federal performance standards and the enforcement of local health codes, filtration is no longer a major concern in patient protection—compliance is almost 100%. The purpose of the filtration is to remove the soft, nonpenetrating, x-ray photons from the x-ray beam (see Chapter 1). These photons would either be absorbed by the overlying tissues or give rise to secondary radiation to the patient and degrade the diagnostic image.

Collimation. The collimation of the x-ray beam limits the size of the area exposed by the primary beam and the amount of scatter produced. The beam size was discussed in Chapter 1 and at present a 2¾-inch circular beam is required. If the size and shape of the x-ray beam were changed to a rectangle that is slightly larger than the film, the volume of tissue exposed could be reduced by more than half (Fig. 4-3). The American Dental Association and the American Academy of Maxillofacial Radiology strongly recommend the use of rectangular collimation (Fig. 4-4).[3]

A **B**

Fig. 4-3. **A,** Open-ended metal rectangular collimator; **B,** Open-ended lead-lined cylinder.

Rectangular collimated beam

Film

Fig. 4-4. Diagram of rectangular collimation.

Timing device. The use of more sensitive x-ray film with extremely short exposure times makes the use of electronic timers imperative. All new x-ray machines come equipped in this manner.

The mechanical timers existing on older machines are inaccurate at short exposure and are usually only calibrated down to 1/4 second. It is impossible to use a mechanical timer with group D and group E films and make accurate exposures. Unfortunately, those that use mechanical timers often compensate for the unavoidable overexposure by underdeveloping and in this way produce a diagnostic radiograph. Mechanical timers should be replaced by the electronic type.

Position-indicating devices. Open-ended, lead-lined (shielded) rectangles (Fig. 4-3, *A*) or cylinders (Fig. 4-3, *B*) are the only type of PIDs that should be used.[3] The use of closed-end pointed cones is contraindicated (see Chapter 1). These cones increase the scattered radiation to the patient because of the interaction of the primary beam with the closed end of the cone (see Fig. 1-18). It is somewhat disconcerting to note that as recently as 1984 a radiation survey of practicing dentists reported that 18% of those surveyed still used the pointed cone.[4] Any existing closed-end pointed cone can be replaced by the recommended types of PIDs.

Receptor (film) holders

Film holders that align the x-ray beam with the film in the patient's mouth should be used.[3] These devices will reduce the possibility of "cone cutting." Some of these devices will also produce rectangular collimation (Fig. 4-5). These film holders should never be held in place for the patient by the operator. Some of the more commonly used film-holding devices are seen in Fig. 7-8.

Film

Decreasing the exposure time by the use of a more sensitive receptor (film, film-screen combinations, xeroradiography) is probably the single most important factor in reducing radiation exposure to the patient. As discussed in Chapter 2, film slower than group D should never be used.[3] Group E film, when compared with group D film, reduces the radiation exposure by 50% (Fig. 4-2). At present the American Dental Association recommends the use of the E speed film. The E film is a major step forward in patient protection. Its use requires an electronic timer and strict adherence to time-temperature processing, because the film has very little leeway for error. The new film has not been universally accepted by practitioners, because there have been claims of lost diagnostic ability. Many recent reports of clinical tests of D versus E film that show that no significant clinical difference exists between the films.[5,6] The possible slight lowering of contrastand loss of detail, which is not apparent without magnification, are far outweighed by the 50% reduction in patient exposure.

Fig. 4-5. Precision device. (Courtesy Isaac Masel Co., Inc., Philadelphia.)

Fig. 4-6. Lead apron with thyroid collar.

Lead aprons and collars

All patients should be draped with a lead apron for all exposures, and a thyroid collar should be used (Fig. 4-6) for intraoral exposures. This rule should be adhered to regardless of the patient's age or the number of films being exposed. The apron should cover the patient from the thyroid to the gonadal area. Leaded aprons with attached cervical (thyroid) shields are available. Separate thyroid collars can be purchased to use with existing lead aprons. The aprons available are usually the equivalent of 0.25 mm lead, relatively light and flexible, and not uncomfortable for the patient. The dose to the gonads is very small during dental exposures but can be reduced even further with the lead apron. The thyroid gland, except with rectangular collimation and more specifically with the bisecting-angle technique, may lie in the path of the primary beam. The dose may be small but can be decreased significantly with the use of the thyroid collar. There is no valid reason not to use the lead apron and collar for every intraoral exposure. Many states have enacted legislation that makes this procedure mandatory.

Lead aprons should not be folded but rather hung up when not in use. Folding will eventually crack the lead and allow leakage.

TECHNIQUE

Retakes

One of the major sources of unnecessary exposure to radiation in the dental office is the retaking of films as a result of poor technique in either the taking or processing of films. Every retake represents an unnecessary doubling of radiation exposure to the patient for that film. It is the obligation of both the dental auxiliary and the dentist to perfect their intraoral technique so that retakes will be unnecessary.

Exposure

Films should be exposed properly. A technique that employs overexposure with underdevelopment subjects the patient to unnecessary radiation. If exposed films come out too dark with time-temperature processing, the exposure time or the kVp, not the developing time, should be reduced. An overexposure and a shortened processing time used to expedite patient treatment is unconscionable in relation to good patient radiation hygiene. An acceptable range of x-ray exposure is seen in Fig. 4-7. The exposures are expressed in milliroentgens and not impulses or seconds. If one knows the output of the dental x-ray machine (mR/sec), then the exposure can be expressed as mR instead of impulses to see whether the exposure falls within the acceptable range. Film packets also come with recommended exposure times, so there is no excuse for overexposure.

Paralleling technique

In addition to the more accurate diagnostic image, the paralleling technique will result in lower dose levels to the thyroid gland and the lens of the eye (see Chapter 7).

"D" Speed Film ★

kVp	Lower Limit	Upper Limit
50	425	575
55	350	500
60	310	440
65	270	400
70	240	350
75	170	260
80	150	230
85	130	200
90	120	180
95	110	160
100	100	140

"E" Speed Film ★ ★

kVp	Lower Limit	Upper Limit
50	220	320
55	190	270
60	165	230
65	140	200
70	120	170
75	100	140
80	90	120
85	80	105
90	70	90
95	60	80
100	50	70

*Exposure Conditions

```
10 mA
 8" S.S.D.
50- 70 kVp - 1.5 mm Al
71-100 kVp - 2.5 mm Al
```

**Exposure Conditions

```
10 mA, 12" S.S.D.
50- 70 kVp - 1.5 mm Al
71-100 kVp - 2.5 mm Al
```

Fig. 4-7. Acceptable range of x-ray exposure. From "Dental Exposure Normalization Technique (DENT) Instruction Manual" developed by the Department of Health and Human Services.

Fig. 4-8. Focal-film distance and tissue volume exposed. Shaded areas represent tissue that is exposed at 8-inch FFD but not in the beam at 16-inch FFD because of the more parallel and less divergent x-rays.

Focal-film distance

Increased FFDs, up to 16 inches, are recommended with the paralleling technique to compensate for the magnification of the image caused by the increased object-film distance (see Chapter 2). Another important advantage of an increased FFD is that there is less total tissue volume in the path of the primary beam at 16 inches than at 8 inches. As the distance increases from 8 to 16 inches (Fig. 4-8), the x-ray beam becomes less divergent and there is less total body area irradiated by the primary beam after it penetrates the skin. The shorter FFD, with a more divergent beam, irradiates a far greater volume of tissue. The diameter of the primary beam is still 2¾ inches at the skin in both cases. The difference is in the beam divergence after the skin entry and film exposure.

Darkroom

Every effort should be made to establish darkroom procedures that will produce films with the maximum diagnostic yield. As previously mentioned, underdevelopment should not compensate for overexposure. There is no excuse for dark room errors that cause retaking of films. This subject is discussed thoroughly in Chapter 6.

Viewing finished radiographs

To get maximum diagnostic yield for the radiation expended, the manner in which radiographs are viewed for interpretation is extremely important. The only proper way to view a radiograph is in front of an illuminator (viewbox), preferably with a variable light source. Using sunlight in front of a window or the lamp on the dental unit is unsatisfactory. The film mount used for the full-mouth survey should cover the entire illuminator, and empty windows in the mount should be covered with an opaque material. This will prevent light that escapes around the periphery or through the mount from distracting the viewer. Ideally, the radiographs should be viewed in a darkened room to avoid excessive reflection.

CLINICAL JUDGMENT

Radiation history

Specific questions regarding the patient's prior exposures should be part of every history. This should include medical, dental, and therapeutic exposures. Questions of this type may help determine whether dental radiographs have been taken recently that might be available and still diagnostically valid. These radiographs also help to give historical data, show previous dental disease, and the results of treatment. Patients may not volunteer such information on their own, thinking it is not important.

Selection criteria

Selection criteria are descriptions of clinical conditions (signs and symptoms) and historical data that identify patients who are most likely to benefit from a particular radiographic examination. They help the dentist to select the patients who need radiographs and determine which radiographs are needed. The final decision rests with the individual dentist and is determined by professional judgment.

Recently published guidelines for the prescription of dental radiographs were developed by an expert panel of dentists sponsored by the Public Health Service.[7] Using these guidelines the dentist can decide when, what type, and how many radiographs should be taken. The practice of taking dental radiographs based on a time interval rather than on patient needs, as determined by the clinical examination and dental history, is not considered an appropriate way to practice dental radiology.[3] The decision regarding the taking of the radiographs should be made by the dentist after examining the patient. There are no "routine dental radiographs." Radiograph needs are not determined by the calendar but rather by evaluating the overall health needs of a patient after a clinical examination and history. This is true for new patients, for those seen emergencies, and for recall visits.

These guidelines, shown in chart form in Fig. 4-9, cover three general categories of patients: those with positive historical findings, patients who are symptomatic, and those who are asymptomatic. Patients are divided into three main categories: (1) children with primary and transitional dentitions, (2) adolescents with permanent dentition, and (3) adults, including dentulous and edentulous patients. Each patient category is further divided into new patient and recall patient categories. In addition, the recall patient category is subdivided into clinical caries or high risk factors for caries, no clinical caries or high risk factors, periodontal disease, and growth and development assessment.

Using these guidelines we can see that all new patients should have a recent full-mouth survey of some type on file before treatment is instituted. The radiographs may have been taken by the present dentist or duplicates of those taken by a previous dentist. The full-mouth survey is essential for case planning, baseline data for future reference, and medicolegal reasons.

Recall radiographs should not be taken on all patients as a matter of routine. As we can see in Fig. 4-9, very few patients need radiographs at 6-month intervals. Caries susceptibility, for example, is a major factor when determining the time frame for recall radiographs. The diagnostic radiographic needs of a decay-prone teenager are quite different from those of a middle-aged periodontal recall patient whose last filling was placed 20 years earlier.

Administrative radiographs

Administrative radiographs can be defined as those required for reasons not related to the patient's immediate health needs. Included in this category would be teaching films, those required by state examination and licensing authorities, and radiographs taken to verify treatment for compensation by insurance companies or other third-party carriers. Radiographs should *never* be taken for administrative reasons. If there is no diagnostic benefit to the patient, the radiograph should not be taken. This is not to say that radiographs should not be submitted to insurance carriers; films taken for diagnostic purposes, or their duplicates, can be submitted because no unnecessary radiation is used. Many states have laws that prohibit the use of administrative radiographs, and the

Patient category	Child	
	Primary dentition *(prior to eruption of first permanent tooth)*	Transitional dentition *(following eruption of first permanent tooth)*
New patient All new patients to assess dental diseases and growth and development	Posterior bitewing examination if proximal surfaces of primary teeth cannot be visualized or probed	Individualized radiographic examination consisting of periapical/occlusal views and posterior bitewings *or* panoramic examination and posterior bitewings
Recall patient Clinical caries or high-risk factors for caries	Posterior bitewing examination at 6-month intervals *or* until no carious lesions are evident	
No clinical caries and no high-risk factors for caries	Posterior bitewing examination at 12- to 24-month intervals if proximal surfaces of primary teeth cannot be visualized or probed	Posterior bitewing examination at 12- to 24-month intervals
Periodontal disease or a history of periodontal treatment	Individualized radiographic examination consisting of selected periapical and/or bitewing radiographs for areas where periodontal disease (other than nonspecific gingivitis) can be demonstrated clinically	
Growth and development assessment	Usually not indicated	Individualized radiographic examination consisting of a periapical/occlusal *or* panoramic examination

Fig. 4-9. Selection criteria chart. (Courtesy Department of Health and Human Services.)

Adolescent	**Adult**	
Permanent dentition *(prior to eruption of third molars)*	Dentulous	Edentulous
Individualized radiographic examination consisting of posterior bitewings and selected periapicals. A full mouth intraoral radiographic examination is appropriate when the patient presents with clinical evidence of generalized dental disease or a history of extensive dental treatment.		Full mouth intraoral radiographic examination *or* panoramic examination
Posterior bitewing examination at 6- to 12-month intervals *or* until no carious lesions are evident	Posterior bitewing examination at 12- to 18-month intervals	Not applicable
Posterior bitewing examination at 18- to 36-month intervals	Posterior bitewing examination at 24- to 36-month intervals	Not applicable
Individualized radiographic examination consisting of selected periapical and/or bitewing radiographs for areas where periodontal disease (other than nonspecific gingivitis) can be demonstrated clinically		Not applicable
Periapical *or* panoramic examination to assess developing third molars	Usually not indicated	Usually not indicated

Fig. 4-9, cont'd. Selection criteria chart. (Courtesy Department of Health and Human Services.)

FDA has recommended that insurance carriers and others refrain from requiring administrative radiographs.[8]

Postoperative radiographs are indicated only when they have diagnostic value, for example, confirming the retrieval of a root tip in surgery or the placement of filling materials in endodontic procedures. The use of radiographs to check the fit, contact, contour, and seating of restorations should be discouraged. This is best done with a mirror, explorer, and floss, thus saving the patient the radiation exposure.

Working films in endodontics, surgery, and restorative post and pin preparations may be necessary for proper treatment, but every effort should be made to keep the number of exposures to a minimum.

OPERATOR DOSAGE AND PROTECTION

As mentioned, of the two concerns in radiation protection, operator and patient, it is much easier to deal with the protection of the operator. The sources of potential exposure to the dental auxiliary are the primary beam, head leakage from the tube, and secondary radiation originating from the patient, x-ray machine, or objects in the operatory. Through the use of careful technique, in a well-designed, well-equipped, and well-monitored office, the occupational exposure to dental auxiliaries and dentists can be kept to a minimum well below the recommended maximum. It should be zero.

Maximum permissible dose

At present the maximum permissible dose (MPD) of whole-body radiation for persons occupationally concerned with ionizing radiation, such as dental auxiliaries and dentists, is 5 rem (0.05 Sv) per year or 100 millirem per week. In addition, the operator should not receive more than 3 rem (0.03 Sv) in any 13-week period. Dental personnel also should not exceed an accumulated lifetime dose of $(N - 18) \times 5$ rem. In this formula, N is the operator's age.

Although 5 rem is the stated MPD at the present time, there is no certainty that this figure will not be revised downward. A recent report by the National Research Council suggested that the MPD might have to be reduced to 1 or 2 rem.[9] Dental auxiliaries and dentists should strive for an occupational dose of zero. It is not difficult to achieve this in an office where there is awareness of radiation hygiene. One should not fear working with x-rays but should be knowledgeable about their use and abuse.

Exposure technique

The dental auxiliary or dentist should never be in the path of the primary beam. Film packets should never be held in the patient's mouth, nor should a drifting tube head be held by the person making the exposure. There are *no exceptions* to this rule. The operator should not make the mistake of saying "I'll

Fig. 4-10. Areas of minimum and maximum scatter during dental x-ray exposure.

just hold the film for the patient this one time." Ideally the operator should be a minimum of 6 feet away from the tube head and behind a suitable barrier when the exposure is made. At 6 feet there will be a minimum occupational exposure that will not exceed the MPD. At 6 feet and behind the barrier, the occupational exposure is zero.

Federal and state regulations require that every x-ray machine be equipped with either a 6-foot retractable exposure cord or a remote switch that will permit such operator positioning. The remote switch is preferable, because it prevents lapses in operator technique. Though not as important as distance and shielding, it is important to know where the areas of minimum scatter are. These areas are at right angles to the x-ray beam and toward the back of the patient (Fig. 4-10). The areas of highest scatter are in back of the tube head and behind the patient. Correct positioning of the operator still necessitates the minimum 6-foot distance or adequate barrier protection.

Radiation monitoring

How can dental auxiliaries and dentists know the amount of occupational exposure of radiation they receive? There are two methods to measure the levels of radiation and potential exposure to concerned personnel. First, a radiation survey can be performed by a health physicist using ionization chambers to determine radiation levels during exposures at all locations in the office. This type of survey checks the reliability of the x-ray machine and protective barriers. It does not monitor the day-by-day activity of the concerned personnel.

Fig. 4-11. Film badge attached to pocket on operator's uniform. (Courtesy ICN Pharmaceuticals, Inc., Cleveland, Ohio.)

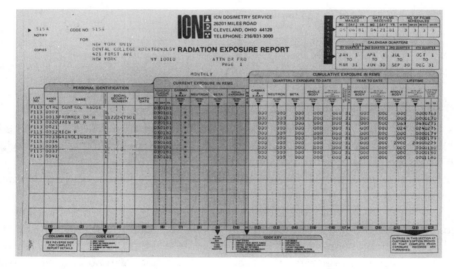

Fig. 4-12. Film badge report. This monthly report gives the current exposure and the cumulative exposure for the listed personnel.

The second method is to have personnel wear pocket dosimeters or film badges. Of the two methods, film badges are less expensive and more widely used. Film badge service is readily available from many radiation survey companies at a nominal monthly cost. The badge (Fig. 4-11) is usually worn for a 3- or 4-week period and contains a film packet, similar to dental film, embossed with the wearer's name and identification number. At the end of the prescribed reporting period, the film packet is returned to the survey company where it is processed; the density on the film is compared with standards and the exposure determined. The report that is returned to the dental office contains not only the exposure for the reporting period but also the accumulated quarterly, yearly, and lifetime exposure of the individual (Fig. 4-12). Using the 100 millirem weekly MPD limit, the dental auxiliary's radiation exposure can easily be evaluated. The film badge should be worn in the office at all times if it is to be an accurate reading of occupational exposure. If clipped to a pocket, it should not be covered with a pen or piece of jewelry that might shield the film. The badge should not be worn outside the office, especially in bright sunlight, and it should be removed if the person being monitored is to have medical or dental x-rays, because it is intended to measure only occupational exposure.

Protective barriers

The walls, floor, and ceiling of the x-ray operatory must be of such construction that the surrounding areas will be shielded from both primary and secondary radiation. This does not mean they must be lead-lined. There are many materials used in construction today that in the proper thickness will provide protective shielding.

Because of the relatively low workload and the low x-ray energies used (65 to 90 kVp), dental offices with concrete or cinder-block walls will have enough inherent shielding in the wall construction materials. Drywall construction, if of proper thickness, is also sufficient for dental shielding.[10]

The shielding or barrier requirements are based on such factors as workload, use and occupancy factors, maximum kilovoltage, and distance from the tube head. The formula W x U x T is used to calculate the guide number. In this formula, W is the workload (in milliampere minutes per week) and U is the use factor. The walls in dental radiography have a higher use factor than the floors or ceiling, because the central ray is never directed straight up or down. T is the occupancy factor, which accounts for whether a person is behind the barrier (1) all the time, as one seated at a desk; (2) sometimes, as in a waiting room; or (3) occasionally, as in a passageway. The guide number is correlated to the proper kVp and distance in reference tables found in Report 35 of the National Committee on Radiation Protection.[11] These tables give the specifications of materials necessary for adequate shielding for the given conditions.

Pregnancy

The pregnant dental auxiliary, as regards occupational exposure, should not be compared with the pregnant patient discussed in Chapter 3. In a well-designed and well-monitored dental office, the occupational exposure, as previously stated, should be zero. Whether one is pregnant or not, zero is still zero, and there is no risk to the fetus. If the auxiliary is apprehensive, a film badge should be worn to document the occupational exposure and allay any fears.

QUALITY ASSURANCE

It is important to establish quality assurance programs in dental offices. to check and monitor x-ray machines, darkroom equipment and procedures, and chairside technique to make sure that ionizing radiation is being used properly

Fig. 4-13. X-ray pulse counter. This instrument is used to check on timer accuracy.

and that the maximum diagnostic yield is being achieved for the energy expended. This is an important part of a radiation protection program. A quality assurance program is easy to establish and maintain. It will reduce exposure to patients and dental personnel and help provide better dental care.

The American Academy of Dental and Maxillofacial Radiology has published an outline of preventive maintenance procedures for radiographic systems.[12] Of the six categories listed in this report, the dental auxiliary, in most offices, would be the person most likely to perform and be responsible for these procedures. The monitoring, calibrating, and inspection of the x-ray generator would be done by a government agency, repair service, or health physicist. The categories in which the auxiliary would be involved include the following:

1. Proper storage and handling of all films, cassettes, screens, grids, and chemicals
2. Posting of current technique charts, including time-temperature for processing, x-ray exposure factors, and x-ray equipment measurements
3. Maintaining proper conditions of processing tanks and automatic processors
4. Maintaining optimal darkroom conditions by periodic checks for light tightness, adequacy of safelighting, cleanliness, and temperature control of the water supply
5. Maintaining the condition of protective devices such as lead aprons, thyroid shields, barriers, and film-holding devices

The quality assurance steps regarding film processing and the darkroom are discussed in detail in Chapter 6.

Periodic testing of the performance of the x-ray machine is essential to a quality assurance program. Some state and local regulatory agencies provide such equipment inspection as part of their registration and licensing programs for x-ray machines. The x-ray machine should be checked for timer accuracy, beam quality, collimation, beam alignment, electrical calibration, barrier adequacy, and tube head stability (Figs. 4-13 to 4-15).

Fig. 4-14. Exposure meter with a digital readout in roentgens.

Fig. 4-15. Survey scatter meter used to check barrier safety.

Another part of a quality control program is the maintenance of high levels of chairside competence. Using programs of self-evaluation, intraoffice peer review, and continuing education, superior levels of chairside technique can be maintained and retakes kept to a minimum.

PATIENT CONCERN AND EDUCATION

It is important for the auxiliary as well as the dentist to understand the patient's concern and possible fear of dental radiographs. Recent years have been marked by a rise of consumerism and an increasing mistrust of health care providers. The media have been replete with stories warning of the danger of medical and dental radiographs.

The dental auxiliary, through knowledge and understanding, must be able to allay fears and explain the necessity of radiographs for proper dental treatment. Many patients will question the auxiliary rather than the dentist about the danger of radiographs. It may be helpful to explain to the patient how essential radiographs are in detecting diseases and planning treatment. Patients can also be made aware of federal and local laws enacted for their protection. Patient educational material, such as the American Dental Association's pamphlet "Dental X-rays: Your Dentist's Advice" or the Food and Drug Administration's "X-rays Get the Picture on Protection," can be placed in the waiting room or given to interested patients.

REFERENCES

1. Performance standards for electronic products: diagnostic x-ray systems and their major components, Fed Register 37:16461, 1972.
2. Brooks SL and Joseph LP: Basic concepts in the selection of patients for dental x-ray examinations, US Department of Health and Human Services (FDA) 85:8249, Sept 1985.
3. Council on Dental Materials, Instruments, and Equipment: Recommendations in radiographic practices: an update, 1988, J Am Dent Assoc 118:115-117, Jan 1989.
4. Kangers GE, Broga DW and Collett WK: Dental radiologic survey of Virginia and Florida, Oral Surg 60(2):225-229, August 1984.
5. Kanter ML, Reiskin AB, and Lurie AG: A clinical comparison of x-ray films for detection of proximal surface caries, J Am Dent Assoc III:967-969, Dec 1985.
6. Kanter ML, et al: Efficacy of dental radiographic practices: options for image receptors, examination selection, and patient selection, J Am Dent Assoc 119:259-268, Aug 1989.
7. Department of Health and Human Services. The selection of patients for x-ray examinations: dental radiographic examinations, Rockville, Md: USGPO, 1987: HHS publication No (FDA) 88-8273.
8. Recommendations on administratively required dental x-ray examinations, Fed Register 45:40976-40979, 1980.
9. The New York Times: Higher cancer risk found in radiation, Dec 20 1989.
10. Macdonald JCF, Reid JA, and Berthoty D: Dry wall construction as a dental radiation barrier, Oral Surg 55:319-326, 1983.
11. National Council on Radiation Protection and Measurements: Dental x-ray protection, Report 35, Washington, D.C., 1970, NCRP Publication.
12. American Academy of Dental Radiology, Quality Assurance Committee: Recommendations for quality assurance in dental radiography, Oral Surg 55:421-426, 1983.

5

Infection control

Infection control has become a major concern in the practice of dentistry. The profession has been or should have been practicing infection control at all times, but the emergence and identification of aquired immunodeficiency syndrome (AIDS) in 1981 has brought the issue to the forefront.[1] Dental personnel have always been at risk for infection from cuts resulting breaks in the skin and contact with body secretions and inhalants. Diseases such as tuberculosis, hepatitis, and herpes have always been a risk for dental workers, but it took the fatal consequences of AIDS to heighten the interest and awareness of the public, the government, and the profession to the importance of infection control in the dental office.

Any comprehensive infection control policy in dentistry must include protocols for radiology, including both chairside technique and darkroom procedures. The fact that radiographic procedures do not involve the aerosol spray produced by the dental handpiece, needles, or the cutting of tissue and the spatter of blood does not exempt radiology from infection control. Infectious disease can be transmitted by the cross-contamination of equipment, supplies, and film packets and cassettes used in the taking or processing of radiographs.

If we understand and practice infection control, we can protect our patients, our fellow workers, and ourselves from harm. Our objective is to be educated so that we can work in a concerned manner but not in a fear-induced hysterical atmosphere. We are educated professionals, and we should act in a manner befitting our profession.

SOURCES OF INFECTION

Through contact with saliva, blood, and nasal and respiratory secretions many instruments and pieces of equipment can become means of transmission of pathogens. A pathogen is a microorganism that can cause disease. Everything that we touch during radiographic procedures is a possible transmitter of pathogens. Our concern then must be with instruments, the x-ray machine, the control panel and exposure switch, clothing, counter tops, the dental chair, the light handle, walls, doorknobs, processors, and patient records. In short, any object that the operator touches after placing the packet in the patient's mouth can be considered contaminated and a source of transmission to the operator or other patients. Looking at the problem the other way, any object that is touched before working in the mouth can be considered a source of transmission to the patient. Thus barriers to the transmission of infective microorganisms must be used. Barriers include gloves, masks, protective eyewear, gowns, and surface coverings. If contamination does occur, as it will in the dental office, then steps must be taken to remove or destroy the pathogen to prevent further transmission.

BARRIERS

Dental personnel should always wear gloves, masks, and protective eyewear when working on patients (Fig. 5-1). Just as there, is no excuse for not standing 6 feet away from the x-ray machine there is no excuse for not protecting oneself from infection. Blood is the most common and easily recognized transmission route of the human immunodeficiency virus (HIV) and the hepatitis B virus (HBV). HIV has been isolated from saliva in some patients. It is true that no cases of transmission of HIV have been documented via the salivary route by casual contact, but this should not serve as an excuse for not wearing gloves, masks, and eyewear. Saliva can be assumed to be contaminated by blood; therefore, there is a potential for transmission.[2]

Any object that the operator touches after placing the film in the patient's mouth must be covered with some removable barrier or disinfected after the patient is dismissed. A good maxim to remember is "the less you touch, the less you have to worry about." Household plastic wrap, plastic bags, or aluminum

Fig. 5-1. Operator making exposure wearing gloves, eyeglasses, and mask.

foil are good barriers. The material should be placed over the chair headrest, the counter top, the arm and PID (cone) of the x-ray machine, control panel, and exposure button (Figs. 5-2 through 5-5). If barriers are not used, these objects must be disinfected after the radiographic procedure is completed. Disinfecting solutions such as Iodophor have the drawback that they may not reach irregular surfaces and have the potential to affect electrical connections (Fig. 5-6).

Fig. 5-2. Plastic wrap covering the yolk of the x-ray machine.

Fig. 5-3. Plastic wrap covering PID (cylinder).

Fig. 5-4. Plastic wrap covering the control panel.

Fig. 5-5. Plastic wrap covering the exposure button.

Fig. 5-6. Disinfecting the x-ray machine with Iodophor.

Sterilization and disinfection

Sterilization produces the total absence of all microorganisms, including spores. The most common methods of sterilization in the dental office are steam autoclaving or the use of the dry heat oven.

Disinfection is the process that results in the absence of pathogenic organisms but not spores. Disinfecting agents are usually employed on surfaces but not on human tissue. Iodophor is an example of a disinfectant commonly used in the dental office. "Cold sterilization," so often used in the dental office, is really a type of disinfection. Some instruments such as plastic film holders, bite blocks, or localizing rings may be damaged by heat sterilization and thus have to be cold sterilized. Most radiographic devices being manufactured today are autoclavable and are clearly marked so.

Antiseptics are agents used on human tissue that are either bacteriostatic or bacteriocidal. In dentistry they are used mainly for handwashing procedures.

In dental radiography, sterilization, disinfection, and antiseptic agents are employed.

Immunization

All dental personnel should have the appropriate immunizations, including that for the hepatitis B virus. There is at present no immunization for the AIDS virus. However, hepatitis B remains a greater risk for dental workers, even though it does not have the certainty of fatal consequences that the AIDS virus does.[3] There has been great concern among dental personnel and in some cases refusal to receive the hepatitis B vaccination; they fear contracting AIDS, since the original vaccine was derived from the serum of people who might have been at high risk for or who had AIDS. These fears have been shown to be unfounded and the new vaccine for hepatitis B (Recombvax HB) is now produced artificially by a recombinant DNA technology and is in no way related to the serum of human donors. All dental personnel should receive the hepatitis B vaccine.

Patient history

Every patient should have a current medical history. This should be done by the dentist at the initial or recall visit using a questionnaire and/or direct questioning of the patient. Information gained by the history will alert the dentist to the presence or history of infectious disease or to those who are in high risk categories. Unfortunately, many potentially infectious patients cannot be identified by history or examination. Thus a rational infection control policy should not distinguish between patient who are known to be infected and those who are not. Every patient should be treated in the same manner and all infection control procedures carried out at all times. There are no exceptions. If there are no exceptions, there can be no surprises.

Film packets

Other than the operator's hands the film packet is the main vector of cross-contamination. The packet remains in the patient's mouth, and when removed it will be coated with saliva or in rare instances with blood. The film packet is handled in the operatory and then transported to the darkroom. There are three methods to prevent transmission of microorganisms by the film packet: (1) sterilization or disinfection of the exposed packet, (2) the use of barrier protection for the packet, and (3) handling technique.

1. Sterilization and disinfection of the film packet is impractical, time consuming, and may degrade or ruin the radiographic image; therefore, these methods are not recommended.[4] Autoclaving or sterilizing by dry heat will destroy the image. Immersing the packet in a disinfecting solution for the required time will result in penetration of the solution to the film emulsion. Thus neither sterilization nor disinfection is recommended.

2. A barrier envelope for sizes #0, 1, and 2 film is now commercially available. The new uncontaminated film packet is placed and sealed in the cellophane-like envelope before to the beginning of the radiographic procedure. All film packets to be used are prepared in this manner. The film packet in the barrier envelope is then exposed and brought to the darkroom. The barrier envelope is then opened, taking care not to touch the film packet, and the film is allowed to drop onto a clean surface. Then with clean hands or new gloves the operator opens the film packets and processes the films (Fig. 5-7).

3. Exposed and hence contaminated film packets should be placed in a receptacle that is outside of the operatory and carried to the darkroom when all the

Fig. 5-7. Barrier pack **A**, with film packet; **B**, in film holder.

Fig. 5-8. Opening contaminated film packet in darkroom.

exposures have been made. The operator should always remember that the gloves being worn are contaminated, so nothing should be touched on the way to the darkroom. Gloves can be changed after the exposures have been made if touching surfaces and objects such as a doorknob is unavoidable. Once the operator is in the darkroom under safelight conditions, the film packets are opened, taking care not to touch the films as they are allowed to drop onto a clean surface. The contaminated gloves are then discarded and the films processed either manually or by automatic processing (Fig. 5-8).

Fig. 5-9. Plastic wrap covering necessary items on work surface.

The use of automatic processors with daylight loaders should be discouraged, because it is almost impossible to avoid contamination because of the tight-fitting hand baffles.[5] It is also very difficult to remove the film from the film packet and to remove one's gloves within the confined space of the daylight loader so that the film can be fed into the uptake.

Processing solutions

The developing and fixing solutions used in the dental darkroom have not been shown to act as sterilizing agents. This is a common misconception. Any contaminated film that is processed will emerge from the processing still contaminated. In automatic processors the rollers and tracts can be contaminated by the film, as can the film hangers in manual processing.

Procedures

1. Cover all appropriate surfaces with plastic wrap or aluminum foil. This should include but not be limited to the PID and arm of the x-ray machine, the control panel and exposure button, and the working surfaces where unexposed films will be placed (Fig. 5-9).
2. Plan in advance. Set out all anticipated supplies (film, film holders, cotton rolls, etc.).
3. Seat the patient and drape in the appropriate manner with the lead apron.
4. Wash hands with antiseptic soap and put on gloves.
5. Make the required exposures, taking care to touch only the covered surfaces. If the procedure is interrupted and you have to leave the room and touch anything (e.g., the telephone), remove your gloves and dispose of them and put on a new pair before resuming work. Each exposed film packet should be wiped dry of saliva and put in a disposable cup that is outside of the operatory.

6. If no other dental procedures are to be done, dismiss the patient. Dispose of all contaminated barriers and supplies in the operatory and then disinfect the appropriate surfaces (e.g., lead apron).
7. Remove contaminated gloves and carry the film container to the darkroom.

Processing

8. Put on new gloves.
9. Under safelight conditions with gloved hands remove the films from the film packet or the film packets from the barrier envelopes by allowing them to drop onto a clean surface. You should not touch the film with your gloved hands. The gloves are considered to be contaminated, since they have touched the film packet.
10. The film packet wrappers and the carrying cup are disposed of and the gloves removed and disposed.
11. The uncontaminated film on the clean surface is then processed either manually or automatically.
12. Since the film is not contaminated, gloves are not indicated for their processing or mounting.

REFERENCES

1. Facts about AIDS for the dental team, ed 2, 1988, Chicago, American Dental Association.
2. Centers for Disease Control: Update: universal precautions for prevention of transmission of human immunodeficiency virus, hepatitis B virus and other blood-borne pathogens in health-care settings, MMWR37, 1988.
3. Klein RS et al: Low occupational risk of human immunodeficiency virus infections among dental professionals, N Engl J Med 318:86-90, 1988.
4. Infection control in the dental office, Eastman Kodak Co, Rochester, NY, 1989.
5. Infection control guidelines for dental radiographic procedures, Newsletter of the American Academy of Oral and Maxillofacial Radiology 17(1):10-11 1990.

6

Film processing—the darkroom

The processing of exposed x-ray film either manually or by automatic processing is an important but often neglected and abused step in the radiographic process. It is at this point in the chain of events that a visible image is produced from which a diagnosis can be made. The x-rays that have penetrated the hard and soft tissue in the patient's mouth have created a latent image on the exposed x-ray film. The processing of this film converts the latent image into a visible image.

The darkroom is one of the areas in a dental office for which the dental auxiliary has complete responsibility. In addition to processing film, the auxiliary must keep the darkroom clean, change solutions regularly, keep accurate records of radiographs processed, and maintain a quality assurance program. Only through meticulous attention to detail can proper darkroom technique be maintained. It is important to realize that the processing of films is vital in the production of the diagnostic radiograph. Errors in the darkroom can easily ruin what would otherwise have been good films, making it necessary to retake the films with the resultant loss of time and increased radiation exposure to the patient. Good chairside radiographic technique must be coupled with good darkroom technique.

The lack of attention to detail and of concern for film processing in many dental offices has been reported in the literature. Biedeman et al, in their study of radiographs submitted to an insurance company for reimbursement, reported that a majority of the radiographs were substandard.[1] Of these substandard radiographs, 20% were judged unsatisfactory because of poor density or improper processing. A study done in Nashville, Tennessee, reported some equally disturbing findings.[2] About 15% of the facilities changed their processing solutions less frequently than recommended, and severe light leaks in the darkroom were found in 10% of the facilities. Over 40% of the darkrooms did not have a thermometer, and over 20% did not have a timer. The most alarming finding was that offices using the sight development techniques showed a much higher mR exposure per film than offices using the time-temperature technique.

It is much easier to prevent darkroom errors than chairside errors. Yet a great many dental patients are receiving excess radiation because of poor processing technique. It is important for the dental auxiliary to have a working knowledge of the chemical reactions taking place in the processing of film. This will help in preventing and correcting errors. To process films without understanding is a "cookbook" technique that leads to errors and to a lack of appreciation for the importance of the processing task. The importance of eliminating darkroom errors, with their increased radiation dose consequences to the patient, should be uppermost in the minds of dentists and auxiliaries.

DESIGN AND REQUIREMENTS OF THE DARKROOM

The darkroom is that room in the dental office set aside for the processing of radiographs. It should be an area used only for that purpose and should not be combined with a dental laboratory or used as a lounge where the coffee pot is kept. The essential requirements and components of a darkroom are that it should be light-tight and have safelight and white light illumination, processing tanks, a thermostatically controlled supply of water, thermometer, timer, film racks, drying racks, and storage space.

Location and size

A properly planned and located darkroom is an important but often overlooked feature in a dental office. Darkrooms are placed in unused spaces, closets, and laboratories without proper concern for the function or importance of the procedures to be done in them.

It is important for dental auxiliaries to have some knowledge of planning, although in most instances they will be working in previously established facilities. However, office renovations and relocation of a practice occur frequently, and the knowledgeable auxiliary can have valuable input in the planning and design of a new office.

The darkroom should be a space unto itself and should be located near the rooms where the x-ray units are placed. This will eliminate the necessity of personnel walking the entire length of the office with wet readings, thereby saving time, eliminating dripping of processing solutions, and reducing office traffic.

The darkroom should be a minimum of 16 square feet (4×4), allowing enough room for one person to work comfortably. The factors that should be considered in determining the space needed are (1) the volume of radiographs to be processed, (2) the number of auxiliaries who will be doing the processing, (3) the type of processing to be done (manual, automatic, or both), and (4) space required for duplicating, drying, and storage.

The walls of the darkroom should be a light color that will reflect the safelighting; darkroom walls do not have to be painted black. The surface of the walls and floor should be of a material that will resist and be cleaned of the processing solutions that will inevitably be spilled or splashed on them.

The darkroom must be completely light-tight so that when the safelight is on it is the only illumination in the darkroom. Because x-ray film is sensitive to white light, any light leaks will fog the film. A fogged film is less diagnostic and in some cases may be completely useless. The easiest way to check for light leaks is to stand in the darkroom in complete darkness; any leaks around the door will be apparent and can be corrected with either black masking tape or weather stripping. The darkroom door should have an inside lock so that the door cannot be opened inadvertently while films are being loaded.

The darkroom should be well ventilated to exhaust the moisture from the drying films and, if a dryer is used, the heat, and to maintain comfortable working conditions. Keeping the darkroom at a reasonable temperature will make it easier to maintain desired processing solution temperatures. It should also be remembered that if unexposed film is stored in the darkroom, high temperatures (above 90° F) will cause film fog.

Lighting

There should be five different light sources in a well-designed darkroom: (1) an illuminating safelight, (2) an overhead white light, (3) a viewing safelight, (4) an x-ray viewbox, and (5) an outside warning light.

Illuminating safelight. When film packets are being opened, when film is being attached to hangers, or when film is being processed, safelight conditions must be maintained. As previously mentioned, white light will fog x-ray film. *Safelight* is any illumination that will not affect the x-ray film (Fig. 6-1). It is a low-intensity light composed of long wavelengths from the orange/red range of the spectrum. X-ray films are more sensitive to the blue/green region of the light spectrum where the wavelengths are relatively short. Red lighting was previously used as safelighting but has been replaced by yellow, because one can see better with yellow lighting. Not all yellow and red lights can be considered safe. The determining factors are the sensitivity to the type of light of the x-ray film being used, as well as the position and intensity of the light source. Usually a 7½- to 10-watt bulb with a yellow filter (e.g., Kodak yellow Morlite M-2) placed 3 to 4 feet from the work surface is used when working with intraoral film. If extraoral screen film is used, a Kodak GBX-2 Safelight Filter with a 15-watt bulb is needed because of the increased sensitivity to light of the film. This filter can also be used for intraoral film.

A simple and reliable test of a safelight is to place a coin on an unwrapped, unexposed piece of dental film under safelight conditions. After 3 minutes of exposure to the safelight, the film is developed. If there is an outline of the coin on the film, the light is not safe; the uncovered part of the film should have been as unaffected as the part covered by the coin (Fig. 6-2).

Panoramic and other extraoral films used with intensifying screens are more sensitive to light than periapical films. As previously mentioned, screen film must be used with a different filter (e.g., Kodak GBX-2). Periapical films can be processed with the GBX filter, or, in offices where both screen and non-

Fig. 6-1. Safelight mounted on wall of darkroom This light is placed 3 to 4 feet from working surface and has a 10-watt bulb with a 6B Wratten filter.

A

B

Fig. 6-2. Coin test for safelighting, **A,** Coin placed on unexposed film under safelight; **B,** Developed film showing outline of coin indicating that safelight intensity is too great and not safe.

screen (periapical) films are used, the darkroom can have two safelights of different intensity.

Overhead white light. There are no special requirements for overhead white light other than providing adequate illumination for the size of the room. The switch for this light should be placed in a position inside the darkroom where it will not be accidentally bumped and turned on, exposing films to white light.

Viewing safelight. Most dental offices will utilize wet readings for emergencies and working films. In these cases it is convenient to have a viewing safelight mounted on the wall behind the processing tanks. In this manner the films can be removed from the fixer after 3 minutes and checked by safelight if they have cleared enough for washing and reading. If a viewing safelight is not located behind the processing tanks, then one would have to hold the wet film up to the overhead safelight with the obvious problem of dripping and staining of the fixer solution. Clearance or the lack of murkiness on the fixed film should never be checked for by holding the film to the overhead white light or the viewbox; in the uncleared state, the film can still be affected by the white light.

X-ray viewbox. It is a great convenience to be able to read the wet films in the darkroom. A proper diagnosis can only be made by having an adequate viewing mechanism. The darkroom should have a viewbox to suit these needs. A diagnosis should not be made by holding a wet radiograph up to the overhead light.

Outside warning light. This light should be wired so that when the safelight is on in the darkroom, the warning light is on outside the darkroom. This is a double-check on the inside lock on the door and helps to prevent entry into the darkroom when safelight precautions are in effect.

Plumbing

The darkroom requires intake lines of hot and cold water with an adequate drainage line. There should be a thermostatically controlled intake valve to maintain constant temperatures of the solutions. The disposal line should be made of materials that will resist the action of the processing chemicals. If automatic processors are going to be used, the rate of flow of the incoming water should be considered in planning darkroom plumbing, because automatic processors have individual requirements.

It is extremely convenient for tank cleaning and solution changing to have a sink with a gooseneck faucet in the darkroom. This is often overlooked in darkroom planning, and one will not be reminded of this until the first time the processing tanks have to be carried to the nearest sink for cleaning and replen-

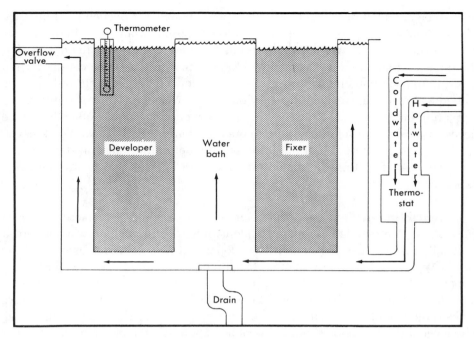

Fig. 6-3. Typical processing tanks in dental office.

ishing. The gooseneck faucet is essential, because a normal-size faucet neck will not allow enough room to place the tanks under the faucet for cleaning.

Contents

Processing tanks. Most dental offices have processing units that contain either 1- or 2-gallon developer and fixer inserts suspended in a tank of running water (Fig. 6-3). The tanks should be made of stainless steel, and the water bath should have a thermostatically controlled flow valve to keep the solutions at the desired temperature. The tank is equipped with a lid that should be kept on at all times. The cover will protect developing films from accidental exposure to white light and prevent oxidation and evaporation of the processing solutions.

Solutions. The developer and fixer solutions are usually supplied as liquid concentrate that have to be diluted. Some commercial services will deliver already prepared solutions in 1-gallon containers. Extra amounts of prepared solutions should be stored either in dark bottles or opaque plastic containers away from heat and light sources.

Under normal working conditions, developer and fixing solutions should be changed at least every 3 to 4 weeks. A normal workload is considered to be 30 intraoral films per day. If many panoramic films are processed, solutions will have to be changed more often, because more chemical is needed per film area. The chemical solutions lose strength when exposed to air and should be replaced even if normal workload minimums have not been met. This means that the times that an office has been closed for vacation still are to be counted when determining solution change timer. If we consider the development of film to be a chemical reaction, we see that every time the developer and fixer solutions affect a film emulsion, the solutions become weakened. In a busy office it may be necessary to change solutions more frequently than every 3 weeks. Weak developer and fixing solutions will not bring out the optimum image on the film and then we are not getting the maximum diagnostic information for the radiation exposure.

Replenishing. Developer and fixer solutions should be replenished on a daily basis. Commercially prepared replenishment solutions are available but it is usually easier to use the standard developer and fixer solutions used to fill the tanks. Approximately 8 ounces of replenishment is required each day for the developer and fixer solutions. If one uses the commercial replenisher then follow the manufacturer's instructions. The replenisher is added in the respective tanks directly to the existing solutions to bring them to the proper fluid level. The level of the solutions should always be kept at the top of the tank to ensure that all the immersed films are totally covered with solution. Water should never be added to the solutions to bring them to tank top level; this dilutes the strength of the chemicals.

The following chart lists the main ingredients of developer and fixer and their function:

Ingredient	Function
Developer	
Elon or Metol and hydroquinone	Reduces the energized silver bromide crystals to silver
Sodium sulfite	Prevents oxidation of developer
Sodium carbonate	Provides alkaline medium and softens gelatin to allow developing agents to reach silver bromide crystals
Potassium bromide	Controls activity of developing agents and prevents chemical fog
Fixer	
Sodium thiosulfate	Removes undeveloped or unexposed silver bromide crystals from the emulsion
Sodium sulfite	Preservative
Potassium aluminum sulfate	Shrinks and hardens gelatin
Acetic acid	Maintains acid medium

Timer and thermometer. No darkroom is complete without a timing device and a thermometer. The most modern radiographic equipment will not produce optimum results if there is no time and temperature control in the darkroom. There is no other correct way to process films. The timer is used to determine the length of time the films stay in the developer solution. This depends on the temperature of the developer—not the temperature of the water in the surrounding tanks or that of the water entering through the flow valve. To de-

Fig. 6-4. Darkroom timer and thermometer, essential parts of time-temperature technique.

termine temperature of the developer, a thermometer must be suspended in the developer tank. Early in the day, developer solutions may be cold or hot, depending on the overnight office temperature. It may take some time for equalization of temperatures between the water tank and the developer tank. That is why the temperature of the developer bath is read, not the temperature of the water entering the surrounding water tank (Fig. 6-4). It is ironic that some dental offices will have thousands of dollars worth of radiographic equipment but will be missing a timer and thermometer whose total costs are about $40.

A time-temperature chart, similar to the following, appears on every package of developer-fixer solution. These charts may vary slightly from manufacturer to manufacturer. A chart like this should be posted in every darkroom.

80° F 2½ minutes in the developer

75° F 3 minutes in the developer

70° F 4 minutes in the developer
⎫
⎬ Optimum
⎭
68° F 4½ minutes in the developer

60° F 6 minutes in the developer

Film hangers. Intraoral film hangers come in various sizes and contain clips for 2 to 20 films. In all cases the films should be unwrapped and attached to the clips without touching the films with one's fingers (Fig. 6-5). This can easily be accomplished by using the wrapping paper in the film packet. The working surface on which the hanger is loaded should be clean and dry to pre-

Fig. 6-5. Placing film on hangers in darkroom under safelight conditions. Note that fingers do not touch film.

vent film staining. Film hangers should be numbered or have the patient's name written on the hanger to avoid mixups. The implications of a film series with the wrong patient's name are obvious. Hangers with defective clips should be discarded because the defective clip can scratch films on adjacent hangers in the solution. Defective clips also lead to lost film in the solutions. The idea that the dental auxiliary will remember which clip is defective and avoid using it is not realistic. If the film hanger is in any way defective, it should be discarded.

Dryer. After films have been washed for 20 to 30 minutes they are ready for drying. This can be accomplished by the use of an x-ray dryer or simply by hanging them on towel racks and letting the films air-dry. In either method the films should not touch one another or they will stick together; separating them will rip the emulsion. The drying racks should be out of the way in a clean room. One of the major objections to laboratory-darkroom combinations is that the dust and dirt of the grinding and polishing done in the laboratory will contaminate the dental films.

THE DEVELOPMENT PROCESS

Procedure

1. Lock the darkroom door from the inside and record the patient's names whose films are to be processed on film hanger.
2. Stir the solutions. This is done to equalize the temperature and the chemical distribution of the processing solutions. Use a different stirring paddle for each solution to prevent cross-contamination. Check the level of solutions and replenish if necessary.
3. Check the temperature and set the timer. The temperature of the developer solution should be checked with an accurate thermometer. Refer to the time temperature chart, which should be posted in the darkroom, and set the time for the desired interval.
4. Turn off the white light and turn on the safelight.
5. Open the film packets and load the film hangers. Work carefully, avoiding finger marks and scratching the film. Be sure the film is securely fastened to film hanger clips.
6. Immerse the film hanger in developer and activate the timer. After immersing the film immediately raise and lower the hanger a few times so that the film surfaces are totally covered by solution. It is preferable to remain in the darkroom while the films are in the developer. It is permissible to leave if the tank lids are securely in place.
7. Remove the film rack from the developer where the timer sounds.
8. Rinse thoroughly for 20 seconds in the water bath.
9. Place the film rack in the fixer solution. Agitate the rack up and down immediately after the initial placement. Films should remain in the fixer for a minimum of 10 minutes for permanent fixation but may be removed after 3 or 4 minutes for use as a wet reading. After doing this, with the tank lids firmly in place, normal lighting can be resumed in the darkroom. It is not necessary to use safelighting after the timer signals that fixation is completed and films are being moved from the fixer to the water bath.
10. Place the films in the running water bath for 20 minutes.
11. Dry the films. Remove the films from the water bath and suspend them from rack holders to dry.

Explanation and discussion

Latent image. Radiographs, after having been exposed, are said to contain a latent image. The silver halide on the radiographic emulsion is energized by the x-ray beam. The pattern of this energizing of the silver halide depends on the density of the objects being radiographed. For instance, the silver halide crystals on the film that lie behind a gold inlay will receive almost no radiation because the dense gold inlay will absorb all the x-ray energy. Silver halide crystals on the film that correspond to an area such as the pulp of the tooth or a

Metallic filling
Pulp
Caries
Dentin
Enamel
Air

1   Latent image;
    energized crystals
    are shaded gray

2   Start of development;
    energized crystals are
    precipitated as free silver
    (black areas)

3   Development complete;
    completely energized silver
    precipitated as black areas

4   Fixer removes unaffected
    crystals, leaving black, white,
    and gray areas

Fig. 6-6. Schematic drawing of x-ray film development.

cavity will receive more radiation energy since these areas are less dense and absorb little x-ray energy (Fig. 6-6).

Developing. Exposed dental film packets that contain a latent image should be processed as soon as possible. In the darkroom under safelight conditions the x-ray films are removed from the packets and placed on film racks. The developer is the first solution into which these film racks are placed. The developer has a pH above 7 and is basic compared with the acidic fixing solution. The developer chemically reduces the energized silver halide crystals by precipitating silver on the film base. This precipitation corresponds to the black (radiolucent) areas on the radiograph. An area of less density, such as the pulp, will allow greater penetration of x-rays; therefore, more x-rays will reach that part of the film. The silver halide crystals will be more greatly energized, and more silver will precipitate to give a black, or radiolucent, outline to the pulp chamber.

This is a chemical reaction. The optimum amount of precipitation of silver for the amount of x-ray energy delivered to the object will take place in a specified amount of time with the developing solution at a certain temperature. This is the basis and importance of the time-temperature technique.

If films are left in the developing solutions too long, more silver will precipitate than was intended and there will be no distinction between dense and less dense structures. A completely overdeveloped film results when all the silver is precipitated by the developer and the film is totally black.

Crystals of silver halide that have received small amounts of radiation will have correspondingly less silver precipitated and will appear gray. The silver halide that was unenergized by radiation, such as the area on the film behind a gold crown, will precipitate no silver and will appear white or radiopaque on the x-ray film.

Washing (stop-bath). The main purpose of washing is to remove the developer from the film so that the development process will be stopped. This also removes the basic developer so that it will not contaminate the acidic fixer. This is usually accomplished by agitating the film rack in a water bath for about 20 seconds. Safelight conditions must be maintained when transferring the films from the developer to the wash tank and then to the fixing solution.

Fixing. The acidic fixing solution removes the unexposed and undeveloped silver halide crystals from the film emulsion and rehardens the emulsion, which has softened during the development process. For permanent fixation the film is kept in the fixing solution for a minimum of 10 minutes. However, films may be removed from the fixing solution after 3 minutes for viewing. This procedure is known as the "wet reading" and is useful when films are needed immediately. For example, a wet reading of a film would be used to check that all the root tip has been removed in an extraction before dismissing the patient. As previously mentioned, a film is ready for a wet reading if it is cleared enough for washing and reading. Clearance or the lack of murkiness is always checked for under safelight conditions.

If these films are to be made part of the patient's permanent record (archival), they should be returned to the fixing solution to complete the required 10 minutes. If this is not done, the films will fade and turn brown in a short time.

Washing and drying. The film is washed for about 20 minutes in the water tank to remove the fixing solution from the emulsion. The film is then dried in a clean, dust-free area.

TIME-TEMPERATURE VERSUS SIGHT DEVELOPMENT

The only correct way to process dental x-ray films is by the time-temperature method described in this chapter. It is the scientific method whereby the optimum information is portrayed on the film. In spite of this, there are still many dental offices that develop x-ray films by sight. The usual technique is to immerse the film hanger in the developer, removing it at frequent intervals to hold it up to the safelight, until fillings or root shapes are visible. At that point the films are washed and placed in the fixer. This is obviously a very inexact, unacceptable technique. The usual reason given for the use of the sight development method is, "We have always done it this way, and it works well." This continual acceptance of lower standards of the quality of radiographs leads dentists and dental auxiliaries to believe that this is the way the radiograph should appear. Sight development is unfair to the patient because it does not provide the maximum amount of diagnostic information for the radiation exposure. To repeat, the time-temperature method, done either manually or by automatic processors, is the only acceptable way to process dental radiographs.

RAPID PROCESSING

Rapid processing of dental radiographs is done with the use of higher solution temperatures, concentrated solutions, agitation of the film, or a combination of these. It is sometimes called "hot processing," referring to the temperature of the solutions. Rapid processing can be done with no increase in radiation to the patient, but the images produced by this technique are not comparable in density and definition to films processed by the standard methods.[3]

The use of regular-strength developing solutions at 92° F with agitation of the film can produce acceptable diagnostic images in less than 1 minute (20 seconds developing, 3 seconds washing, and 30 seconds fixing). There are also concentrated processing solutions available that can be used at room temperature. The increased chemical activity of these solutions makes the rapid processing possible. Some of these solutions use a two-bath technique, developer

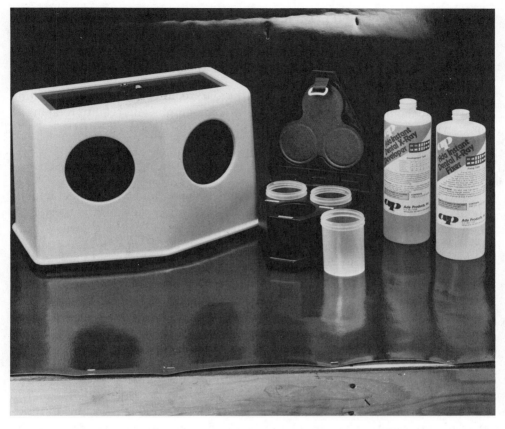

Fig. 6-7. Rapid processing system *(left to right)* light-tight working area with hand baffle, solution receptacles, processing chemicals. (Courtesy: Ada Products/Block Professional Dental Products Company.)

and fixer; others use a single-bath technique or monobath that contains the developer and the fixer (Fig. 6-7).

Rapid processing can be a very helpful technique with endodontic working films and postoperative films in oral surgery where a high degree of definition is not essential. It should not be used for routine processing of films.

EXTRAORAL AND PANORAMIC FILMS

These films are processed in the same manner as intraoral films using the time-temperature technique with the same solutions. As mentioned earlier, the only precaution that must be taken is to check the intensity of the safelight. Those extraoral films that are used in combination with intensifying screens (screen films) are more sensitive to light than nonscreen films. Darkroom illumination that may be safe for intraoral films may adversely affect screen films. The safety of the light can be checked by using the coin test discussed earlier.

CARE AND MAINTENANCE OF THE DARKROOM

Although the maintenance of a darkroom may seem like a housekeeping chore, it is really a means of ensuring quality control in the darkroom. Maintenance should be likened to our regard for sterility to avoid contamination and subsequent infection. Contaminants in the darkroom or other errors resulting from sloppy techniques may ruin diagnostic radiographs and require retaking of films, with an unnecessary increase in the patient's radiation burden.

Cleanliness

The working surface, where films are stripped and placed on hangers, should always be clean and dry. Developer, fixer, and water are the most common stains. Drying films should not be placed above the working surface without catch pans. If the working surface is made of formica, it can easily be cleaned with a mild detergent. Film hangers should be clear and dry when loading films. Hangers used for wet readings are the most likely ones to be insufficiently washed and contain residual fixer that can stain the next film. Hangers should be washed after each use and clean, dry hangers should always be used.

Processing tanks should be cleaned thoroughly when solutions are changed. This not only means the insert tanks that hold the developer and fixer but also the water reservoir. The water tank will accumulate sludge and algae, especially under the metallic lip and in the overflow tube. A bland detergent can be used or preferably one of the tank cleaners made specifically for this purpose. It is in this routine cleaning of the tanks that one appreciates the sink and gooseneck faucet in the darkroom.

Solutions

Solutions should be brought to the optimal temperature at the beginning of the working day and kept at that temperature by the thermostatic control on the mixing valve.

Tanks should be kept full by the use of replenishers, not by adding water, since such an addition will dilute the concentration and weaken the solutions. If the tanks are not kept full, the films or portions of the films on the top clips of the film rack may not be fully immersed in solution and will not be developed.

As mentioned before, both the developer and fixer solutions should be changed at least every 3 to 4 weeks regardless of use. In some practices with heavy film volume, it may be necessary to change solutions as often as once a week.

The lids of the processing tanks should always be closed when the tanks are not in use to prevent oxidation and weakening of the solutions.

Record keeping

Two types of records are important in the darkroom. The first is the supply inventory, including the date of the next scheduled solution change. It is helpful to have the date of the next scheduled solution change posted in a prominent place.

Film identifications are the second type of records that are important in the darkroom; accurate records are essential when processing radiographs. The patient's name, the number of films, the number or letter of the rack the films were placed on, and the date should be recorded. This will eliminate the likelihood of lost films and mixed x-ray series.

Silver retrieval and scrap foil

There are two sources of silver retrieval in the dental office: (1) the old and no longer needed or unusable processed radiographs and (2) the exhausted fixer solution.[4]

Silver can be recovered from the processed radiographs by ashing the film above the melting point of silver. The economic benefit of this endeavor is limited—a pound of radiographs is worth less than $25.

Residual silver can be retrieved from the fixer by either chemical precipitation or electrolysis. There is no residual silver in the developer solution.

Electrolysis units that can be inserted into dental processing tanks can be purchased for under $100. At the present price, silver retrieval may not be worth the investment in equipment and time but local health codes may prohibit the dumping of fixer solution into the local sewer system because of the silver content making the silver retrieval a mandatory process.

The lead foil inserts of film packets can be saved and sold for scrap. Since the foil is very thin, it will take a great amount of it to accumulate a salvageable lot.

AUTOMATIC PROCESSING

In recent years automatic dental x-ray film-processing units have become available and more popular. They are not an essential component of a darkroom but a substitute for manual time-temperature processing. Their major advantage is the maintenance of standardized procedure; these units provide solutions of proper strength, correct temperature, and regulated processing time. In short, they provide automated time-temperature processing. Other advantages of the units are the time saved and the increased volume of films that can be processed when compared to the manual method. However, these units are costly, they still require maintenance, and a quality control program. Some offices that use automatic processing still maintain a backup system of manual processing tanks.

Daylight loader

Drying element

Film

Film

Film exit

Developing
solution

Fixing
solution

Water
wash

Drying
element

Fig. 6-8. Diagram of automatic film processor.

The typical automatic processor has three solutions—developer, fixer, and wash—and a drying chamber (Fig. 6-8). A transport system of either rollers or tracks driven by either gears, belts, or chains move the film from solution to solution and then into the drying chamber. A finished film is produced in 4 to 7 minutes and some units have the capacity to do faster processing by elevating the temperature of the solutions.

Automatic processors vary in the size film they can accept, their safelight and plumbing requirements, and whether or not they have automatic replenishment. Freestanding units are not connected to water and waste lines and may be kept in the operatory as films are fed into the unit through a daylight loader.

Size of film. Some units will accept only periapical and bite-wing size film (#0, #1, #2, #3), while others can accommodate all sizes including 8- × 10-inch and 5 x 12 or 6 x 12 inch panoramic film (Fig. 6-9).

Safelight. Some processors must be located in the darkroom because safelight procedures are required for stripping and insertion of the film. Units with daylight loaders do not have to be in the darkroom as they have light-tight baffles into which the hands are placed while stripping and inserting the film into the rollers (Fig. 6-10).

Plumbing. If there is a constant flow of water in the wash chamber, then plumbing is required. This arrangement is more desirable than a freestanding chamber where the water level may drop and constant change is necessary.

Fig. 6-9. Automatic processor being used in darkroom under safelight conditions.

Fig. 6-10. Automatic processor with daylight loader being used in operatory.

Automatic replenishment. The more sophisticated processors maintain solution concentration and levels by automatic replenishment. Each time a piece of film is fed into the unit, a few drops of fixer and developer are automatically added to the baths to maintain solution strength.

Care and maintenance

Automatic processors need daily or weekly cleaning, depending on the volume of films processed. The rollers should be cleaned at the beginning of the day by running an extra oral-size film or cleanup film that is made specially for cleaning through the rollers. This will remove any residual gelatin or dirt from the rollers. The rollers should be removed weekly from the processor and soaked in a water bath for about 20 minutes.

Solution levels should be checked at the beginning of every day and replenished when necessary. Quality assurance checks are also necessary. The processors are only as good as the care given them by their operators.

Technique is also important and cannot be neglected just because the machine runs automatically. Films should not be fed into the rollers too quickly. There should be at least a 10-second interval between films on the same track. This will prevent the overlapping of films in the processing and the chemicals not being able to reach the overlapped portions of the film. In fact, it is good practice to alternate tracks when feeding the film into the processor. Carelessness can lead to feeding the film with the black paper or lead foil still attached. Not only does this ruin the film, but also the foil and paper may stick to the rollers, ruining subsequent films.

QUALITY ASSURANCE

An effective quality assurance (QA) policy for the darkroom is the prime responsibility of the dental auxiliary. A quality assurance program in the darkroom is as important as, and is much easier to conduct, than the QA monitoring of the x-ray machine. There should be monthly checks on the safelighting, light-tightness of the darkroom, and the accuracy of the timer and thermometer. There should be daily monitoring of the cleanliness of counter tops, condition of the film hangers, and the strength and level of the processing solutions.[5]

The chemical strength and the level of the processing solutions in both the manual tanks and the automatic processor must be monitored on a daily basis. This is the most critical part of a QA program. Processing solutions should be changed at a maximum of every 3 to 4 weeks. There are better ways to determine when solutions should be changed than just using the calendar.

An easy way to check solution strength in an office, although admittedly a rough estimate, is by comparison to a standard (Fig. 6-11). A processed periapical film of ideal density should be kept taped to the darkroom viewbox for comparison of densities with the films that are processed daily. A lessening of the

Fig. 6-11. Reference film used to check solution strength by comparing densities.

Fig. 6-12. Step wedge and film prior to exposure.

film density in the processed film would indicate a weakened solution and signal the need for solution change. Do not wait until the films become undiagnostic to change solutions; this type of reasoning offers little comfort to the last patient before the solution change, whose films become useless.

A better and more scientific way to check the strength of solutions is to make a test exposure at the beginning of every working day. This test exposure is done through a step wedge or a predetermined density (Fig. 6-12). The film is then processed and compared with standard film densities. In the device shown in Fig. 6-13, the processed film is placed in a slot and the numbered densities are moved until a visual match of densities is achieved. If the test densities are too light, the solutions are either weak or cold. If the densities are too dark, the solutions are either too concentrated or too warm. In either case it is a "no go" situation, and processing cannot begin until the situation is remedied.

Fig. 6-13. A, Dental radiographic normalizing and monitoring device; **B,** Test film inserted beneath copper plate and exposure made; **C,** Processed test film *(arrow)* inserted in device and being compared to numbered densities.

The strength of the fixer can be gauged by noting the length of time needed to clear films. Fresh, full-strength fixer will clear films in 2 to 3 minutes. If clearing requires over 4 minutes, the fixing solution is weakened and should be changed.

Unexposed and unprocessed film should be stored in a cool dry location. High storage temperatures will increase film fog. Film should be stored at temperatures between 50° F and 70° F, and between 40% and 60% relative humidity.[6] Film should be used before the date of expiration that is clearly marked on each box, and film boxes should be placed on the shelf so that the oldest film is in the front.

DUPLICATING RADIOGRAPHS

In recent years, with the increase in dental insurance programs and a more mobile patient population, there are many occasions in which it may be necessary to provide radiographs to insurance carriers or forward films to the patient's new dentist. Coupled with this has been the increase in the number of dental malpractice suits for which the defendant-dentist's records are of utmost importance. Radiographs are an essential part, if not the most important, of these records. The use of radiographic duplicating film can satisfy requests for radiographs and still maintain the integrity of office records. Radiographs should never leave the dental office without having been duplicated. There should be no exception to this rule. We live in a litigenous society, and we must protect ourselves.

Duplication of radiographs is a relatively easy process that requires only a few additions to normal darkroom equipment, namely duplicating film, appropriate-sized film hangers, a light source (ultraviolet is preferable), and a photographic printing frame (Fig. 6-14). Duplicating devices are also commercially available that can duplicate all film sizes or just one film (Fig. 6-15, *B*).

Fig. 6-14. "Home made" set up for radiographic duplication.

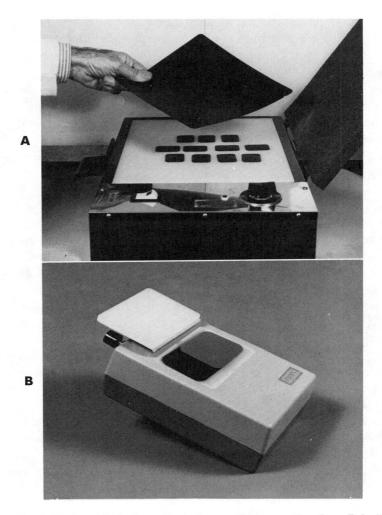

Fig. 6-15. A and **B,** Radiographic duplicators. (**B** courtesy: Rinn Corp., Elgin, Ill.)

Radiographic duplicating film is readily available from dental supply firms and is supplied in 8- x 10-inch or 5- x 12-inch sheets as well as individual periapical-sized duplicating film. The photographic emulsion is coated on only one side of the film. Under safelight conditions that emulsion side will appear dull when compared with the shiny, nonemulsion side. The duplicating film is a direct positive film; therefore if more film density is required (darker film), the exposure time is shortened. Conversely, if decreased film density is desired (lighter film), the exposure time is increased. This is just the opposite in time requirements for exposing dental films to x-rays. The key to remember is to think the opposite of what you would logically do. Duplicating films do not have an orientation dot as standard intraoral films do, and so the films must be labeled right and left.

Fig. 6-16. Maxillary molar radiograph that has been fogged. Note lack of definition and contrast.

Procedure

Under safelight conditions the radiographs to be duplicated are placed in close contact with the emulsion side of the duplicating film. A photographic printing frame is ideal for this, because it has a rigid frame with a glass front that will hold the original radiograph against the duplicating film. This frame is placed on a tabletop and exposed to a light source for 4 to 5 seconds with the light source about 2 feet from the film. Since intensities of light sources may vary from office to office, trial exposure should be made to standardize time and light source distance. After the exposure is made, the duplicating film is processed on an 8- x 10-inch film rack in the same manner that x-rays are, using either manual or automatic technique. There is no limit to the number of times an original radiograph can be copied. Close positive contact between the radiograph and the duplicating film is essential, or a blurred image will occur. The glass top of the printing frame should provide this contact. Films should always be removed from the mounts so that tight contact can be achieved.

COMMON DARKROOM ERRORS

The following are the most common errors made in the darkroom.

Fogged film (Fig. 6-16)**.** Fogged film will have an overall gray appearance because of diminished contrast. This can be caused by light leaks in the darkroom, improper safelighting, or improper film storage.

Remedy. Safelight conditions can be tested with a coin (see p. 88). All doors should be checked for possible leaks, and old film should be used first.

Underdeveloped film (Fig. 6-17)**.** Underdeveloped film will be light in appearance and will not contain all the diagnostic information that is possible. This results when the optimum amount of silver has not been precipitated because of weak developing solutions, insufficient developing time, or developing solutions that are too cold.

Fig. 6-17. Underdeveloped film.

Fig. 6-18. Overdeveloped film.

Remedy. The developer and fixing solutions should be changed every 3 to 4 weeks, and the time-temperature method should be used. That is, the temperature of the developer should be checked before immersing the films in the solution, and the timer should be set for the appropriate time as given in the manufacturer's specifications, referring to density comparison standard mounted on the viewbox. Daily QA checks should be performed to determine solution strength.

Overdeveloped film (Fig. 6-18). Overdeveloped film may vary from dark to totally black, depending on the degree of overdevelopment. This type of film is of no diagnostic value. It results when too much silver has been precipitated on the film base, and in the case of the totally black film all the silver from the silver bromide has been precipitated. This error can be caused by hot developing solutions or prolonged developing time.

Remedy. The time-temperature method of processing should always be used. The timer being used should have a bell or buzzer that will ring when the developing time has elapsed. This will enable the dental auxiliary to leave the darkroom while the films are being processed. Without the bell the dental auxiliary may be distracted by other duties and forget to remove the films from the developer at the proper time. Perform daily QA checks on solution strength.

Developer cutoff (Fig. 6-19). Cutoff film will show a straight radiopaque border on what was the upper edge of the top film on the processing rack. Actually, this represents an underveloped area of the film. When the solutions are allowed to deplete in the processing tanks, the films on the top positions on the

Fig. 6-19. Radiographs with developer cutoff.

Fig. 6-20. Clear film. This can result from excessive washing or fixing or an unexposed film.

racks may not be covered by solution when the racks are placed in the tanks. This error should be differentiated from cone cutting, which may give a curved radiopaque border. In cone cutting the film portion is unexposed; in developer cutoff the film portion is undeveloped.

Remedy. The dental auxiliary should always check to see that the processing tanks are full. If the level of solutions has dropped, water should not be added; this will only dilute the solution and result in underdeveloped films. The proper replenisher solutions should be added to maintain the desired level.

Clear films (Fig. 6-20). Films are clear because the entire emulsion has been washed off. This occurs when films that have had complete fixation are left in running water baths for 24 to 48 hours. This type of film is identical to an un-

Fig. 6-21. Stained radiograph.

exposed film that is developed and processed. With the unexposed film the fixer removes all the unaffected silver bromide crystals.

Remedy. Films should never be left in water baths overnight. Processing should be complete before one leaves the office. Films should not be left in the fixer overnight or for prolonged periods beyond the recommended 10 minutes; the fixer will lighten and finally remove the image. It is a common misapprehension that films cannot be overfixed.

Stained films (Fig. 6-21). If the working surface in the darkroom is wet and dirty, films can be stained either before or after processing. There is no excuse for this error.

Remedy. Darkroom work surfaces must be kept clean and dry.

Discolored films. Films that have not had adequate fixation (approximately twice the developing time) will turn brown after a period of time and will be useless as part of the patient's permanent record.

Remedy. All films must have adequate fixation time (10 minutes). All wet readings should be returned to the fixation tank after the patient has been treated.

Torn emulsion (Fig. 6-22). If films that are drying are allowed to touch and overlap, they will stick together. In separating the films the emulsions are usually torn off the film base in the overlapped area, rendering the film nondiagnostic.

Remedy. Film racks should be checked to be sure that drying films from different racks are not touching.

Scratched films (Fig. 6-23). A radiopaque line on a film is usually an artifact caused by scratching the emulsion on the film base in the processing of films.

Fig. 6-22. Radiograph with torn emulsion.

Fig. 6-23. Scratched radiograph.

Fig. 6-24. Fluoride artifact. Operator's fingertip contaminated by fluoride touched film when stripping and placing film on hanger.

Most often it is caused by putting a second film rack into a tank that already contains a film rack. It can also be caused by fingernails scratching the film while unpacking the film and placing it on a rack.

Remedy. When film racks are put into the processing solution, care should be taken to avoid touching those already immersed. Any film racks should be discarded if they have sharp edges or broken clips that could scratch other films.

Lost film in tanks. If films are not firmly clipped onto the hangers, they may fall off in any of the three processing baths. A lost film necessitates a retake or results in a "wet elbow" in an attempt to retrieve it from the processing solution.

Remedy. All films should be checked to see that they are clipped securely to the hangers before processing.

Fluoride artifacts (Fig. 6-24). Some fluorides, especially stannous fluoride, will produce black marks on radiographs.

Fig. 6-25. Reticulation.

Remedy. After working with fluoride, the auxiliary should wash hands thoroughly with soap and a weak acid, such as vinegar or lemon juice, before handling films in the darkroom.

Reticulation (Fig. 6-25). If developing is done at an elevated temperature and then the film is placed in a cold water bath, the sudden change in temperature will cause the swollen emulsion to shrink rapidly and give the image a wrinkled appearance called "reticulation."

Remedy. Sharp contrasts in temperatures between processing and the water bath should be avoided.

Air bubbles (Fig. 6-26). If air bubbles are trapped on the film as it is placed in the processing solutions, the chemicals will be prevented from affecting the emulsion in that area.

Remedy. The film hangers should always be agitated when they are placed in the processing solutions to dislodge any trapped air bubbles.

Static marks (Fig. 6-27). Static electricity can be produced when intraoral film packets are forcefully opened in the darkroom. With the introduction of new film packets this is not common for intraoral film. The static electricity will produce multiple black linear streaks on the radiograph. The same effect occurs much more frequently on extraoral films. With these films it may happen when removing the piece of film from a full box—the sliding of the film out of the

Fig. 6-26. Artifact caused by air bubbles trapped on the film preventing processing solution from touching film in the area.

Fig. 6-27. Periapical radiograph with static marks.

tightly packed box may produce the static electricity. It also may be produced when loading and unloading flexible cassettes in panoramic machines as the film is slid in or out between the intensifying screens. Static electricity may also be created by walking around a carpeted office. If the auxiliary does not touch a conductive object before unwrapping the film, the charge marks may result. Static electricity is seen most often on cold, dry days.

Remedy. The operator should ground himself or herself by touching any conductive object in the darkroom before handling film and should avoid friction of any kind against the film that will produce static electricity.

Daylight loaders—light leaks (Fig. 6-28). Film fog, a ruined film, or unusual artifacts can be caused by removing one's hands from the baffle (see Fig. 6-10) before the film has completely entered the processor.

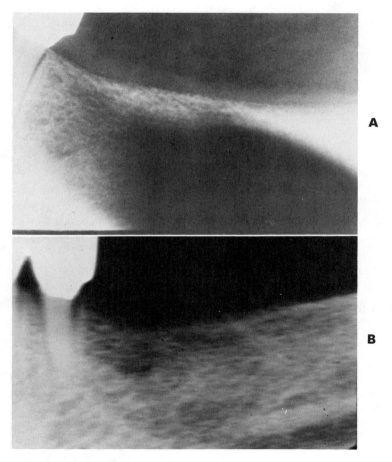

Fig. 6-28. A, Artifact caused by light leak in daylight loader resembling a large pathologic area in bone; **B,** Normal radiograph of same area.

Fig. 6-29. Bands of stain *(arrows)* from dirty rollers of automatic processor.

Fig. 6-30. Overlapped films during automatic processing.

Remedy. The operator's hands must be kept on the film until it has been completely taken up by the rollers. The material that makes up the baffle should fit tightly around the hands. Rips and tears should be repaired immediately and stretched elastic replaced. It is a good idea to remove wristwatches and bracelets, because they tend to tear the baffle material.

Automatic processing

Dirty rollers (Fig. 6-29). If the rollers are not cleaned periodically, radiolucent bands will appear on the finished film.

Remedy. Rollers should be cleaned periodically by removing them and soaking in accordance with the manufacturer's recommendations. A piece of ex traoral film should be run through at the beginning of every work day.

Overlapped films (Fig. 6-30). If the films are fed into the processor too quickly, they overlap and the processing solutions will be unable to reach the emulsion.

Remedy. The operator should wait 10 seconds before putting a following film into each processing tract.

REFERENCES

1. Beideman RW and others: A study to develop a rating system and evaluate dental radiographs submitted to a third party carrier, J Am Dent Assoc 89:1010, Nov 1976.
2. Bureau of Radiological Health: Nashville dental project: an educational approach for voluntary improvement of radiographic practice, U.S. Department of Health, Education, and Welfare Publication (FDA) 76-8011, Rockville, MD, July 1975.
3. Alcox RW and Jameson WR: Rapid dental x-ray film processing for selected procedures, J Am Dent Assoc 78:517, March 1969.
4. Mirada FJ and others: Economics of electrolytic recovery of silver from radiographic fixing solutions, J Am Dent Assoc 100:523, April 1980.
5. Recommendations for quality assurance in dental radiography, Oral Surg 53:4, 1983.
6. Quality assurance in dental radiography: Health Sciences Division, Eastman Kodak Co, Rochester, NY, 1989.

7

Intraoral radiographic technique: the paralleling method

THE FULL-MOUTH SURVEY

The full-mouth radiographic survey is one of the cornerstones of a complete oral diagnosis. No dental examination or treatment plan can be considered complete without current or valid radiographs. The full-mouth survey is a difficult procedure to do correctly and requires time and meticulous attention to detail. It bears with it the responsibility of exposing the patient to the least amount of ionizing radiation to obtain the maximum diagnostic yield. Unnecessary radiographs or those of poor quality that have no diagnostic value do not serve the patient's needs and only add to the patient's radiation burden. Whether the radiographs are taken by the dentist or the dental auxiliary is not important, as long as the same standards are maintained.

The full-mouth radiographic survey is usually composed of 14 or more periapical films and, where possible, four posterior bite-wing films. This text will discuss a 15-periapical and four bite-wing film technique, using two films for the maxillary central and lateral incisors. A 14-periapical film series would use one film projection for these four teeth. Some series of more than 15 periapical films include distal maxillary molar projections, vertical bite-wings, anterior bite-wings, and individual radiographs using #1 size film of the six maxillary and four mandibular anterior teeth.

The number of radiographs in a full-mouth survey can be modified to include extra or fewer projections, depending on the size of the patient's mouth or tooth position. In all cases the minimum number of films that satisfy the diagnostic requirements of a full-mouth survey should be used. Film mounts are available in combinations of number and size of film. The radiographic survey should not be determined by the film mount available but by the diagnostic needs of the patient. The recommended film projections (Fig. 7-1) are as follows.

Maxillary	Mandibular	Bite-wing
Right and left central and lateral incisors	Central and lateral incisors	Right and left premolars
Right and left canines	Right and left canines	Right and left molars
Right and left premolars	Right and left premolars	
Right and left molars	Right and left molars	

Fig. 7-1. A 19-film full-mouth survey.

A periapical film shows the entire tooth from occlusal edge to apex and 2 to 3 mm of periapical bone. It is this film that is necessary to diagnose normal or pathologic conditions of root, bone, and tooth formation and eruption (Fig. 7-2).

The bite-wing film can be taken only if there are opposing teeth so that the film can be held in position by their occluding surfaces. This film projection shows the upper and lower teeth in occlusion. Only the crown of the teeth are seen. It is used for detecting interproximal decay, periodontal bone loss, recurrent decay under restorations, and the fit of metallic restorations (Fig. 7-3). Bite-wing films can be taken of the anterior teeth but are usually unnecessary if the paralleling method is used.

The full-mouth survey will show all of the teeth in the mandible and maxilla as well as the surrounding bone. Each tooth can be seen at least twice in the survey; that is, the maxillary second premolar can be seen on the premolar periapical film and on the premolar bite-wing film. Some teeth may be seen in three or four views. This gives the diagnostician an opportunity to view the

Fig. 7-2. Periapical radiograph of the maxillary central incisor area. Note that the entire tooth and surrounding periapical bone are visualized.

Fig. 7-3. Top, Bite-wing radiograph. Note that only the crowns, alveolar ridge, and a small part of the roots of opposing teeth are seen; **Bottom,** Types of bite-wing films. Left-vertical, middle-long posterior, and right-standard.

tooth from different radiographic angles and eliminates the possibility of artifact that could be mistaken for caries or other pathologic conditions.

All the teeth-bearing areas of the jaws are covered in a full-mouth survey. However, one is not just radiographing the teeth: A clinically edentulous area may have residual root tips, unerupted teeth, or other pathologic conditions in the bone. One should not assume that because there are no teeth present everything is all right. The full complement of periapical films should be taken on all patients.

Pedodontic full-mouth series

Depending on the child's age and the size of the child's mouth, the composition of the full-mouth series may vary.

Up to the age of 5 it is necessary to use the pedodontic-size film #0 for anterior, posterior, and bite-wing projections. The full-mouth series at this age will be 12 films: three maxillary anterior films, three mandibular anterior films, four mandibular and maxillary premolar-molar projections, and two bite-wing projections. The size of the child's mouth does not necessitate separate premolar and molar films. For the same reason, only one bite-wing film is taken on each side.

In the 6- to 9-year-old group the pedodontic film or narrow adult film size #1 can be used for anterior projections, since the child's arch shape at this age can still be very narrow. For the posterior projections, adult size #2, narrow adult, or pedodontic film is used, depending on the size of the arch. At this age two posterior periapical films in each quadrant are taken, since the 6-year molars have erupted and the dental arch has lengthened. One bite-wing film on each side is also used.

After age 9 the full adult series is taken, using the narrow adult film where necessary. These age guidelines are flexible and depend on the growth and development of the child. As a rule it is best to use the largest film size that can be comfortably accommodated by the patient (Fig. 7-4).

In the pedodontic series the chair position, film placement, point of entry, and vertical and horizontal angulations follow the same rules as in the adult series.

CRITERIA FOR INTRAORAL RADIOGRAPHS

The criteria for judging whether a single radiograph or a full-mouth survey is diagnostically acceptable are:
1. The radiograph should show proper definition and detail and a degree of density and contrast so that all structures can be easily delineated.
2. The structures should not be distorted either by elongation or by foreshortening.

Fig. 7-4. Full-mouth pedodontic survey of a 9-year-old patient.

3. The radiograph should show the teeth from the occlusal or incisal edges to 2 to 3 mm beyond their apices.
4. In a full-mouth survey, the entire alveolar processes of the mandible and maxilla must be seen—as far distal as the tuberosity in the maxilla and the beginning of the ascending ramus in the mandible.
5. All interproximal surfaces of the teeth should be seen without overlapping, providing the teeth are not overlapped in the mouth.
6. The x-ray beam should be centered on the film so there are no unexposed parts of the film ("cone cuts," or "collimator cutoff").
7. The radiograph should not be cracked or bent or have any other artifacts.
8. The radiograph should be processed properly (see Chapter 6).

In a single radiograph, if these criteria have not been met and the radiograph is not diagnostic, then it must be retaken. In a full-mouth survey, those areas and structures that do not appear on the primary film may be seen on adjacent films in the series. Although a technically perfect full-mouth survey is the ideal, retakes should not be done unless judged necessary for proper diagnosis.

These criteria should be used to evaluate radiographs taken by dentists and dental auxiliaries as part of a quality assurance program. This can be accomplished by either self-analysis and criticism of one's work or by peer review. In this manner, technical errors will be corrected and high-quality diagnostic radiographs produced.

PARALLELING TECHNIQUE

The basic principle of the paralleling technique for intraoral periapical films is that the film packet and the long axis of the tooth being radiographed must be parallel to each other, and the central ray of the x-ray beam must be directed perpendicular to both (see Fig. 2-10). To accomplish this parallelism, the object-film distance must be increased. This distance can be sizable in some areas, such as the maxillary molar projection where the film may have to be held at the midline of the palate to achieve this parallelism.

The increased object-film distance will result in loss of image sharpness and thus is compensated for by using a 16-inch FFD (Fig. 7-5).

Unfortunately, the paralleling technique has too often been called the *long cone* technique. This has led to emphasis being placed on the length of the PID rather than on the parallel relationship of the object and the film. Better names for this technique are the *extension paralleling* or *right-angle technique,* both of which stress the important components of the technique.

Advantages and disadvantages of the paralleling technique compared with the bisecting technique

When comparing the paralleling technique with the bisecting technique, it should be pointed out that there is a general consensus that the paralleling method is the one of choice.[1] The paralleling technique produces better diagnostic images, less exposure to critical organs such as the thyroid and lens of

Fig. 7-5. Bisecting, 8-inch focal-film distance technique and paralleling 16-inch extended-cone technique. Note superimposition of zygomatic arch on apices of maxillary molar in bisecting technique. (Courtesy Rinn Corp., Elgin, Ill.)

the eye, and is easier to standardize and execute than the bisecting technique. This text takes the position that the paralleling technique is the method of choice.

Advantages. The major advantage of the paralleling technique is that when performed correctly the image formed on the film will have both linear and dimensional accuracy and the diagnosis made from the radiograph will be more valid. The key terms are dimensional accuracy and *dimensional distortion*.

The bisecting technique will correctly represent the teeth linearly but will have dimensional distortion. The bisecting technique projects the images and surrounding structures on the film in a true linear relationship without elongation or foreshortening. When radiographed with the bisecting technique, performed ideally, a tooth 22 mm in length will be seen on the radiograph as 22 mm long. The teeth and bone, however, are three-dimensional objects, and although their overall length may be recorded accurately, the relationship of one part of the tooth to another will be dimensionally distorted (Fig. 7-6). Those parts of the tooth that lie farthest from the film, for example, the buccal plate of

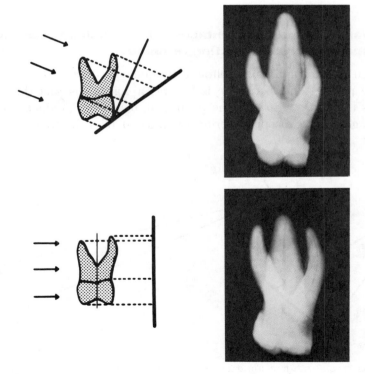

Fig. 7-6. Radiographs of maxillary molar taken with bisecting technique *(top)* and the paralleling technique *(bottom)*. (Courtesy Rinn Corp., Elgin, Ill.)

bone and buccal roots, will be foreshortened although their lingual linear counterparts will not. The classic clinical example of this is comparing the length of the buccal roots to palatal roots in maxillary first molars. Those clinicians who have used the bisecting technique for many years may really come to believe that the buccal roots are much shorter than they really are because of dimensional distortions. One may argue that this may not be clinically important, except in an initial endodontic measurement, but when this distortion is applied to periodontal evaluation of alveolar bone levels, the clinical importance becomes apparent (Fig. 7-7). In the bisecting technique the image of the buccal bone level is figuratively added to the palatal bone height to give a distorted image. A diagnosis and treatment plan could then be made of adequate bone for restorations, fixed splinting, and so forth on distorted radiograph images.

With the paralleling technique, it is possible to diagnose and evaluate car-

Fig. 7-7. Radiographs of the same area, **A,** taken with the paralleling technique; and **B,** the bisecting technique. Note the difference in alveolar bone height as indicated by arrows.

ies and alveolar bone height accurately on all radiographs and not rely on the bite-wing projections, as the users of the bisecting technique do. It is interesting to note that bite-wing projections in both techniques are paralleling films.

In the bisecting technique the radiopaque image of the zygomatic arch is often superimposed on the apices of the maxillary molars, making diagnosis very difficult, if not impossible. This superimposition is understandable because the point of entry of the central ray for molar projections is along the zygomatic arch.

In the paralleling technique there is no superimposition, since the central ray, which is perpendicular to the long axis of the molars, enters below the level of the zygomatic arch (see Fig. 7-5). Also, in the paralleling technique the vertical angulation of the primary beam is rarely more than plus or minus 10 degrees, compared to vertical angulation of plus 40 to 50 degrees in the bisecting technique. The lack of extreme vertical angulation reduces the exposure to the thyroid gland and lens of the eye as they no longer lie in the path of the primary beam. The literature reports thyroid exposure of 25 mR for a full-mouth survey using the paralleling technique compared with 60 mR for the bisecting technique.[2] In addition, the 16-inch focal-film distance employed with the paralleling technique reduces the volume of tissue irradiated when compared to the 8-inch focal-film distance used in bisecting (see Fig. 4-8).

The paralleling technique is easier to standardize than the bisecting technique, and serial comparison radiographs of the same area have greater validity. This is especially important in evaluating alveolar bone levels of periodontal patients at recall examinations.

If a film-holding device is used that has a localizing ring, the patient does not have to be positioned so that the occlusal plane of the jaw being radiographed is parallel to the floor. This is especially helpful in contour chairs or where patients are treated in the supine position. In both these instances it is very difficult to position the patient with the occlusal plane parallel to the floor.

Disadvantages. One of the objections most often raised in regard to the paralleling technique, is the difficulty in placing and the degree of discomfort caused by the devices used to hold the film parallel to the long axis of the tooth. For patients with small mouths, for children, and for patients with low palatal vaults this may present some problems, but the more adept one becomes with the technique, the less these problems are a factor.

It is said that paralleling is more difficult to learn and takes clinically longer to do. Experience with novice students has proved this to be incorrect.[3] At the least, the time element is the same, and learning the paralleling technique is as easy or easier than learning the bisecting technique.

Objections have been raised to the "long bulky" 16-inch position indicating device that is used in the paralleling technique. It is claimed that it is difficult to work with in small operatories. The difference is 8 inches, and in a well designed office this cannot be a factor, This objection has no validity in the newer x-ray machines with the extended FFD within the tube head (see Fig. 2-7).

Another supposed disadvantage of the paralleling technique is that with the 16-inch FFD, longer exposure times are necessary and there may be greater chance of patient movement. With the use of faster film this is no longer true. We are comparing exposure times of ⅕ versus ⅘ second (inverse square law), and the difference in the possible patient movement within these time frames is not significant. Previously, with the use of slower film, the possibility of patient movement with a 4-second exposure, compared with a 1-second exposure, was greater and the objection was valid.

EXPOSURE ROUTINE

Regardless of which technique is used, there are certain basic rules that must be followed regarding barrier technique, preparation of the patient, and radiation hygiene. A routine should be developed so that mistakes that necessitate retaking of films can be avoided. Retaking a radiograph because of an error by an operator adds unnecessarily to the patient's radiation burden.

The patient should be seated comfortably in the chair, with the back well supported and the head positioned so that the jaw can be radiographed correctly. Except when localizing rings are used, the occlusal plane of the jaw being radiographed must be parallel to the floor when it is in the open position.

The patient should remove any nonfixed prosthetic appliances from his mouth, as well as eyeglasses from his face. Failure to do this is a common error. Glass and any metallic frame are radiopaque and may be superimposed on the film in the maxillary canine and premolar areas.

The patient should be draped with a lead apron. This is done routinely on all patients, for a single film as well as the full-mouth series. The x-ray machine should then be turned on and the desired kilovoltage and milliamperage selected.

The infection control procedures outlined in Chapter 5 should be followed. Most dental offices will have a semiautomatic, lead film dispenser in each operatory. This enables the operator to withdraw one film at a time. Care should be taken not to touch the dispenser with the gloved hand after it has been in the patient's mouth. If a dispenser is to be used it should be activated with the upper part of the arm or elbow. The exposed films are placed in a paper cup within a lead receptacle. If there is no lead dispenser, the desired number of films, as well as additional supplies such as bite-wing tabs and bite blocks, should be brought near the operatory at this time.

If there are no lead film dispensers and no exposed film receptacles, both the exposed and unexposed films must be kept out of the room where the x-ray machine is being used. Many diagnostic dental films are fogged by secondary radiation and thus made unacceptable because they are left on the bracket table in the dental operatory when other films are being exposed. Again, poor technique on the part of the operator leads to film retakes and unnecessary exposure for the patient.

One of the more important general principles of intraoral radiographs is to have the positioned film in the patient's mouth for as short a time as possible. This will decrease the likelihood of gagging and patient movement. The desired exposure time on the machine should always be set before placing the film in the patient's mouth. Many seconds can be wasted in consulting exposure charts and setting the timing dial while the film is in the patient's mouth.

While the exposure is made from the required 6-foot distance, the patient should be watched. In this way, if the patient moves, the error will be detected and a retake film can be done immediately. A properly designed office will permit this observation from behind a suitable barrier.

After the exposure has been made, the film is removed from the patient's mouth, dried of saliva, and placed in the exposed film receptacle.

Some definite order should be followed for a full-mouth series of radiographs. Skipping from area to area without a set pattern will always result in an omitted film. It is appropriate to start with the maxillary central incisor film which is probably the easiest to position and the easiest for the patient to tolerate. One should never start with the maxillary molar film, because this is the projection most likely to excite the gag reflex; once the reflex is excited, the patient may gag on films that could normally be tolerated. After starting with the maxillary central incisor, the maxillary canine, premolar, and molar are radiographed in that order. The opposite side of the maxilla is then radiographed. It is poor technique to radiograph left canine, right canine, left premolar, and so forth. This necessitates moving the tube head constantly from one side of the patient to the other and usually results in an omitted film.

The bite-wing films are taken after maxillary periapicals, since the same head position and occlusal plane orientation are used. The mandibular periapical films are then taken in the same order as the maxillary films.

Film holders

The use of film holders is strongly recommended. In the paralleling technique the film packet must be held in its proper position by one of a variety of film-holding devices all serving one purpose: to position the film parallel to the long axis of the tooth. Some of the devices, such as hemostats, Stabes, XCP, Precision, and Intrax holders are pictured in Fig. 7-8. Localizing rings align the PID with the film in both the horizontal and vertical planes and help to reduce the incidence of cone cutting. The localizing rings are a great aid in some of the contour dental chairs in which it may be difficult to position the patient so that the occlusal plane is parallel to the floor. As long as the open-ended PID can be brought into flat contact with the localizing ring, strict adherence to occlusal plane orientation is not necessary.

Film holders are either disposable (e.g., styrofoam bite blocks) or nondisposable (e.g., XCP). The nondisposable film holders must be sterilized and not just disinfected.[5] As described in Chapter 5, the accepted methods of sterilization include steam autoclave, dry heat, chemical vapors, and ethylene oxide.[6]

Fig. 7-8. Film-holding (receptor) devices for use in paralleling technique. Left to right: XCP, Stabe, Intrax, Precision paralleling device, hemostat, Snap-A-Ray.

Some holding devices have plastic or vinyl parts that are not considered autoclavable.

METHOD

There are six factors that must be considered in any periapical projection: exposure time, chair position, film position and placement, point of entry of the beam, vertical angulation, and horizontal angulation.

Exposure time

Exposure time is determined by the area being radiographed, the film speed, kVp, milliamperage, and FFD. Exposure charts are readily available, and most x-ray film packages contain them. It is customary to post such a chart near the machine so that exposure times need not be committed to memory. The timer should always be set before placing the film in the patient's mouth.

Chair position—occlusal and sagittal plane orientations

The patient is positioned so that when the mouth is open and the film packet is in position, the occlusal plane of the jaw being radiographed is parallel to the floor. In the maxilla this plane corresponds to the ala-tragus line on the face. When the maxilla is radiographed, the headrest is positioned high on the

Fig. 7-9. Proper patient position for maxillary periapical radiographs and bite-wing films. Note that occlusal plane of maxillary teeth, or ala-tragus line, is parallel to the floor.

Fig. 7-10. Proper patient position for mandibular periapical radiographs. Note that when mouth is open occlusal plane of lower teeth is parallel to the floor.

Fig. 7-11. Proper patient position for orientation of sagittal plane of head perpendicular to the floor.

back of the patient's head, forcing the chin down (Fig. 7-9). When the mandible is filmed, the headrest is placed below the occipital eminence, in what would be the normal dental chair position (Fig. 7-10). For both upper and lower jaws the patient's head is positioned so that the sagittal plane is perpendicular to the floor (Fig. 7-11).

Film position

The film packet is held with its long dimension vertical for anterior projections and horizontal for posterior periapical and bite-wing projections. The edge of the film should always extend evenly either ⅛ inch below (maxillary) or above (mandibular) the occlusal plane. This ensures adequate film at the apical area to record the image. The film should be placed in the patient's mouth so that the mounting orientation button is toward the occlusal surface (Fig. 7-12). This helps in mounting and precludes the possibility of the dots being superimposed over the apex of a tooth. The film is held in position by the patient with a bite block or other film-holding device.

Point of entry

The point of entry is the anatomic position on the patient's face at which the central ray of the x-ray beam is aimed. It corresponds to the middle of the film packet in the patient's mouth. The operator should know these anatomic points but should also align the beam with the film as viewed in the patient's mouth. The localizing ring, when used, will determine the point of entry by its predetermined relationship to the film packet.

Fig. 7-12. Placement of film holding device in patient's mouth by operator. Note that correct side of film packet faces tube head and mounting dot is toward incisal edge.

Vertical angulation

In the paralleling technique the vertical angulation is set to make the central ray perpendicular to the film. In the bisecting technique (see Chapter 8), the vertical angulation is determined by the bisection of the angle. The vertical angulations for the bisecting technique given in this text and elsewhere should be used only as guide angles. With ideal film positioning these angles can be strictly adhered to. However, not all mouths will allow this type of film positioning. Some mouths have crowded arches, misplaced teeth, and tight muscle attachments. In these cases the bisection of the film-tooth angle will result in different vertical angulations than the ones listed. Vertical angulation of the x-ray beam is set according to the dial on the side of the tube head (Fig. 7-13).

Horizontal angulation

The central ray is directed so that it is perpendicular to the film in the horizontal plane. It can also be said that the central ray is directed through the interproximal spaces to avoid overlapping of structures. It may be easier for the operator to sight on the horizontal axis of the tube head and make this parallel to the film in the horizontal plane.

Fig. 7-13. Photograph of tube head of x-ray machine, with arrow pointing to setting for vertical angulation.

THE FULL-MOUTH SERIES

Maxillary central and lateral incisors (Fig. 7-14)

Chair position. The maxillary occlusal plane is positioned parallel to the floor, and the sagittal plane of the patient's face is perpendicular to the floor.

Film position. The film is held vertically and positioned in the palate away from the lingual surfaces of the teeth so that the long axis of the film packet will be parallel to the long axis of the teeth. The center of the film packet is between the central and lateral incisors. The film is positioned in the palate so that the entire length of the teeth will be shown. This parallel placement of the film is held in position by one of the devices previously mentioned.

Point of entry. The central ray is directed at the center of the film. If a localizing ring is used, the open face of the PID contacts the ring; this will then determine the point of entry and vertical and horizontal angulation of the x-ray beam.

B

A

C

Fig. 7-14. Maxillary central and lateral incisors. **A,** Film holder and position indicating device (PID); **B,** Radiograph; **C,** Diagram.

Fig. 7-15. Right and left maxillary central and lateral incisors. **A,** Film holding device and PID. **B,** Radiograph.

Vertical angulation. The central ray is perpendicular to the film packet.

Horizontal angulation. The central ray is perpendicular to the film in the horizontal plane.

If one film is to be used for the maxillary right and left central and lateral incisors, the center of the film is placed between the central incisors and the central ray is directed perpendicular to the center of the film packet (Fig. 7-15).

Maxillary canines (Fig. 7-16)

Chair position. The maxillary occlusal plane is parallel to the floor, and the sagittal plane of the patient's face is perpendicular to the floor.

Film position. The film is held vertically, away from the lingual surface of the canine, and parallel to its long axis. The center of the film packet is behind the canine and is positioned in the palate so that the entire length of the canine will be shown. The film packet is held in position by a holding device.

Fig. 7-16. Maxillary canine. **A,** Film holding device and PID; **B,** Radiograph; **C,** Diagram.

Point of entry. The central ray is directed at the center of the film packet, or if a localizing ring is used, it is brought into flat contact with the open-ended PID.

Vertical angulation. The central ray is perpendicular to the film packet.

Horizontal angulation. The central ray is perpendicular to the film in the horizontal plane.

Fig. 7-17. Maxillary premolars. **A,** Film holding device and PID; **B,** Radiograph; **C,** Diagram.

Maxillary premolars (Fig. 7-17)

Chair position. The maxillary occlusal plane is parallel to the floor, and the sagittal plane of the patient's face is perpendicular to the floor.

Film position. The film is held horizontally and positioned away from the lingual surfaces of the premolar so that its long axis is parallel to the long axis of the premolar. In the maxillary premolar and molar region this may position the film in the middle of the palate. The center of the film aligns with the second premolar. The packet is positioned in the palate so that the entire length of the teeth will be shown on the film. The packet is held in position by a holding device.

Point of entry. The central ray is directed at the center of the film, or the localizing ring is brought into flat contact with the open-ended PID.

Vertical angulation. The central ray is perpendicular to the film.

Horizontal angulation. The central ray is perpendicular to the film in the horizontal plane.

Fig. 7-18. Maxillary molars. **A,** Film holding device and PID; **B,** Radiograph; **C,** Diagram.

Maxillary molars (Fig. 7-18)

Chair position. The maxillary occlusal plane is positioned parallel to the floor, and the sagittal plane of the patient's face is perpendicular to the floor.

Film position. The film is held horizontally and positioned away from the lingual surfaces of the molars so that the long axis of the film will lie parallel to the long axes of the molars. The center of the film packet aligns to the middle of the second molar, and the packet is positioned in the palate so the entire length of the teeth will be shown. The film packet is held in position by a holding device.

Point of entry. The central ray is directed at the center of the film, or the localizing ring is brought into flat contact with the open-ended PID.

Vertical angulation. The central ray is perpendicular to the film.

Horizontal angulation. The central ray is perpendicular to the film in the horizontal plane.

BITE-WING FILMS

The technique for bite-wing films is the same in the paralleling and bisecting angle technique except for the use of the 16-inch FFD and thus increased exposure time. Bite-wing films are always parallel films, no matter what technique is used for the periapical films. The film is positioned by the bite tab parallel to the crowns of both upper and lower teeth, and the central ray is directed perpendicular to the film.

Premolar and molar bite-wing projections (Fig. 7-19)

Chair position. The maxillary occlusal plane is positioned parallel to the floor, and the sagittal plane of the patient's face is perpendicular to the floor.

Film position. When the premolars are radiographed, the bite tab is placed on the occlusal surfaces of the first and second mandibular premolars. This will depress the film packet into the floor of the mouth. While the operator holds the tab down with thumb and forefinger, the patient is instructed to bite on the tab. The operator should be sure that the patient is biting on the back teeth and not just bringing the incisors together. If the back teeth are not moved to centric occlusion, the film packet will not be secure and may move and will not be oriented correctly. The procedure for radiographing the molars is the same as that previously mentioned, except that the bite tab is centered over the occlusal surface of the second molar.

Point of entry. The central ray is directed at the bite-wing tab, which is held in position by the patient's teeth. If a localizing ring and film holder are used then the open end of the PID is placed against the ring.

Vertical angulation. The central ray is perpendicular to the film.

Horizontal angulation. Horizontal angulation is a critical factor in the bite-wing film, and utmost attention should be paid to horizontal position. An overlapping image on the bite-wing film is useless. The central ray should be perpendicular to the film packet in the horizontal plane and should go through the contact points of the premolars or molars.

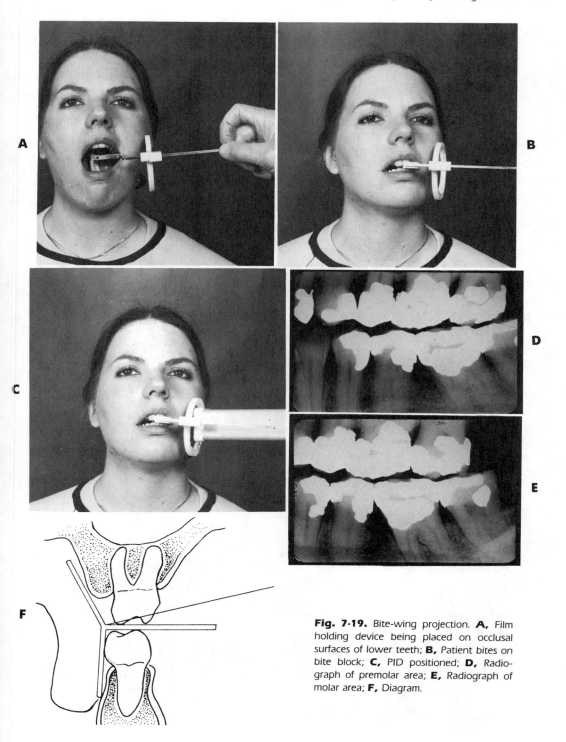

Fig. 7-19. Bite-wing projection. **A,** Film holding device being placed on occlusal surfaces of lower teeth; **B,** Patient bites on bite block; **C,** PID positioned; **D,** Radiograph of premolar area; **E,** Radiograph of molar area; **F,** Diagram.

VERTICAL BITE-WINGS (FIG. 7-20)

Vertical bite-wings are used when the desired area would not be seen on the film with normal bite-wing placement; this could be the case in advanced bone loss or root caries. The film is placed in the patient's mouth with the longer side vertically positioned. All other exposure factors remain the same. It is necessary to use the paste-on tabs and not the loops or the preformed bite-wing packets in this technique. The vertical bite-wing can be used in a posterior or anterior region.

Fig. 7-20. Vertical bite-wing. **A,** Posterior film position; **B,** Posterior radiograph; **C,** Anterior film position; **D,** Anterior radiograph.

Mandibular incisors (Fig. 7-21)

Chair position. The patient is positioned so that when the mouth is open the mandibular occlusal plane is parallel to the floor and the sagittal plane of the patient's face is perpendicular to the floor.

Film position. The film is held vertically and positioned away from the lingual surfaces of the incisors so that the long axis of the film will be parallel to the long axes of the incisors. The center of the packet is positioned at the midline so that all four incisors will appear on the film. The film is depressed into the floor of the mouth so that the entire length of the teeth will be shown. It may be necessary to displace the tongue distally as well as to depress the floor of the mouth to achieve this. The film packet is held in position by a holding device.

Point of entry. The central ray is directed at the center of the film, or the localizing ring is brought into flat contact with the open-ended PID.

Vertical angulation. The central ray is perpendicular to the film.

Horizontal angulation. The central ray is perpendicular to the film in the horizontal plane.

A

B

C

Fig. 7-21. Mandibular incisors. **A,** Film holding device and PID; **B,** Radiograph; **C,** Diagram.

Mandibular canines (Fig. 7-22)

Chair position. The patient is positioned so that when the mouth is open the mandibular occlusal plane is parallel to the floor and the sagittal plane of the patient's face is perpendicular to the floor.

Film position. The film is held vertically and positioned away from the lingual surface of the canine so that its long axis will be parallel to that of the canine. The packet is positioned so that the canine will be in the center of the film. The packet is depressed into the floor of the mouth so that the entire length of the tooth will be shown on the film. The packet is held in position by a holding device.

Point of entry. The central ray is directed at the center of the film, or the localizing ring is brought into flat contact with the open-ended PID.

Vertical angulation. The central ray is perpendicular to the film.

Horizontal angulation. The central ray is perpendicular to the film in the horizontal plane.

A

B

C

Fig. 7-22. Mandibular canine. **A,** Film holding device and PID; **B,** Radiograph; **C,** Diagram.

Mandibular premolars (Fig. 7-23)

Chair position

The patient is positioned so that when the mouth is open the mandibular occlusal plane is parallel to the floor and the sagittal plane of the patient's face is perpendicular to the floor.

Film position. The film is held horizontally and positioned so that it is parallel to the long axes of the premolar. The object-film distance in both the mandibular premolar and molar regions is almost minimal since the anatomy allows the film to be positioned very close to the tooth and still be parallel. The second premolar is centered behind the center of the film packet. The packet is depressed into the floor of the mouth so that the entire length of the teeth will show on the film. The film is held in position by a holding device.

Point of entry. The central ray is directed at the center of the film, or if a localizing ring is used, it is brought into flat contact with the open-ended PID.

Vertical angulation. The central ray is directed perpendicular to the film.

Horizontal angulation. The central ray is perpendicular to the film in the horizontal plane.

Fig. 7-23. Mandibular premolar. **A,** Film holding device and PID; **B,** Radiograph; **C,** Diagram.

Mandibular molars (Fig. 7-24)

Chair position. The patient is positioned so that when the mouth is open the mandibular occlusal plane is parallel to the floor and the sagittal plane of the patient's face is perpendicular to the floor.

Film position. The film is held horizontally and positioned lingually to the molar so that the long axis of the film is parallel to the long axes of the molars. The film is centered behind the second molar and depressed into the floor of the mouth so that the entire length of the teeth will appear on the film. The packet is held in position by a holding device.

Point of entry. The central ray is directed at the center of the film, or if a localizing ring is used, it is brought into flat contact with the open-ended PID.

Vertical angulation. The central ray is directed perpendicular to the film.

Horizontal angulation. The central ray is perpendicular to the film in the horizontal plane.

A

B

C

Fig. 7-24. Mandibular molars. **A,** Film holding device and PID; **B,** Radiograph; **C,** Diagram.

COMMON ERRORS

All the errors mentioned and illustrated in this chapter are also possible in the bisecting technique, but the incidence differs. Whereas elongation and fore-shortening are the most common bisecting errors, they are not that common in the paralleling technique. The most common error in the paralleling technique, even with the use of positioning devices, is in film placement. If the film packet and film holder are not placed correctly in the patient's mouth, the paralleling technique will not work. The most common error is to not place the film packet deep enough in the floor of the mouth or high enough in the palate, thus cutting off the apices of the teeth.

With the use of the localizing ring, which is aligned with the center of the film packet, cone cutting can be practically eliminated.

Occlusal plane and sagittal plane orientation of the patient's head is not important if the localizing ring on the film-holding device is used, as long as the open end of the PID is brought into flat contact with the localizing ring.

Horizontal overlapping of the images is also eliminated with the proper use of the positioning device and localizing ring.

The rest of the errors mentioned in this chapter (i.e., film reversal, over-bending, crescent marks, overexposing and underexposing, double exposure, and failure to remove dental appliances) are all possible with the bisecting technique, and their remedies are the same.

Cone cutting (collimator cutoff) (Fig. 7-25). An unexposed area on the radiograph occurs when the x-ray beam is not centered on the film packet. This is called cone cutting and is caused by improper x-ray beam film alignment.

Fig. 7-25. Collimator cutoff ("cone cutting"). Central ray positioned too far distal.

Remedy. The central ray of the x-ray beam should be carefully aligned with the center of the film packet. With circular collimation the aperture of the diaphragm allows for a beam diameter, measured at the face, of 2¾ inches. Size #2 adult film is 1¼ × 1⅝ inches, which leaves almost ½-inch leeway for error in all directions. It is not sufficient to identify collimator cutoff; it should be analyzed to pinpoint the error. If it is always the distal part of a radiograph in a projection that is cut off, then the point of entry must be moved mesially. A localizing ring, with a film-holding device, will align the beam and the film and eliminate collimator cutoff.

Film reversal (Fig. 7-26). Film reversal is sometimes referred to as the "herringbone effect" because the herringbone pattern embossed on the lead foil backing is transferred to the processed, reversed radiograph. The "herringbone" light film results from placing the film packet backward in the patient's mouth. The x-rays are attenuated by the lead foil before striking the film. The pattern embossed in the lead that appears on the film distinguishes this light film from other underexposure errors.

Remedy. The front and back of the film packet should be noted. Some manufacturers color code or change the texture of the back of the packet. One should develop the habit of looking for these aids.

Fig. 7-26. Film reversal. Film packet placed in mouth with the wrong side toward the tube.

Film placement (Fig. 7-27). The film has been poorly positioned if the whole tooth does not show on the film and the image is not elongated; there is no film behind the apex of the tooth to record the image.

Remedy. Only ⅛ inch of film should project above or below the occlusal or incisal edges of the teeth. If a bite block is used, the teeth being radiographed must be biting firmly on the block.

Fig. 7-27. A, Nondiagnostic due to poor film-packet placement. Note that apices of teeth are not seen; **B,** Poor film placement. Note how much film is visible above occlusal plane of tooth.

Fig. 7-28. Overlapped images.

Fig. 7-29. A, Proper; and **B,** improper horizontal angulation of x-ray beam.

Overlapping (Figs. 7-28 and 7-29). Overlapping of the images of the teeth will result if the central ray is not perpendicular to the film and teeth in the horizontal plane.

Remedy. The film should be aligned with some part of the tube head that is perpendicular to the central ray. There is usually a horizontal bar with the manufacturer's name on it. Standing in front of the patient, the operator should retract the patient's cheek and check the horizontal alignment. As in cone cutting, a positioning device with a localizing ring can be used to prevent overlapping. If the film is placed parallel to the teeth, the localizing ring will align the beam perpendicular to the film.

Crescent marks and bent films (Figs. 7-30 and 7-31). Black crescent-shaped marks can be caused by excessive bending of the film packet, which cracks the emulsion. The crescent marks show when the film is developed. A film may be overbent to such a degree that the x-rays will not strike it at all.

Remedy. Films can be made more pliable by rolling them slightly against one's index finger, which also may allow them to fit better in the patient's mouth. Films should not be bent to adapt to anatomic surfaces. X-rays travel in straight lines; they do not turn corners to expose bent films.

Fig. 7-30. Black line due to cracking of film emulsion.

Fig. 7-31. Result of overbending film packet. Note upper-right corner,

Fig. 7-32. Underexposed radiograph.

Light films (Fig. 7-32). Light films or films that do not have enough density can result from underexposure or underdevelopment, assuming that the proper kVp has been used. If not enough kVp has been used, the dental structures will be underpenetrated and the film, although light, will not differentiate structures of different density.

Remedy. For underexposure all settings on the machine should be checked before making an exposure (mA, time, kVp).

A very common error that leads to underexposure is unwittingly increasing the FFD by failing to bring the open end of the PID close to the patient's face. The exposure times are calculated for an FFD that assumes a PID placement close to the face. If the PID is carelessly positioned away from the face, the inverse square law will intensify the error, not just by the increased distance but the square of that distance (Fig. 7-33). For a discussion of underdevelopment, see Chapter 6.

Dark film (Fig. 7-34). Dark film is caused by overexposure or overdevelopment, the reverse causes of light films. The length of the PID prevents the possibility of decreased FFD. If a film is overpenetrated, it will be black and none of the dental structures will show or they will be difficult to differentiate.

Remedy. For overexposure all settings on the control panel should be checked before making an exposure. For a discussion of overdevelopment, see Chapter 6.

A   **B**

Fig. 7-33. A and **B.** Light film will be caused by increased focal-film distance without compensatory increase in exposure time. Note distance between patient's face and PID,

Fig. 7-34. Overexposed radiograph.

Fig. 7-35. Double exposure on radiograph.

Double exposure (Fig. 7-35). A double exposure results from using the same film packet twice. This is an unforgivable error and indicates lack of attention to detail.

Remedy. After the film packet has been exposed, it should be placed in a lead receptacle. The exposed and unexposed films should never be kept on the same shelf.

Blurred images (Fig. 7-36). Blurred images are the result of either patient, film, or tube head movement during the exposure.

Remedy. Tube heads and arms should be adjusted to prevent vibration and drifting. In most states this is a serious health code violation. Good chairside technique will prevent film and patient movement.

Failure to remove dental appliances or facial jewelry (Figs. 7-37 and 7-38).
If dental appliances or pieces of facial jewelry are not removed, the metallic portions will be superimposed on the tooth structure.

Remedy. It should be a part of the work routine to have patients remove all dentures, nose jewelry, and eyeglasses. For panoramic and extraoral projections patients must also remove earrings, hearing aids, and hair clips.

Fig. 7-36. Blurred image caused by patient movement.

Fig. 7-37. Patient's partial denture was not removed.

Fig. 7-38. Facial jewelry (nose ring) was not removed.

Poor bite-wings (Fig. 7-39)

The three most common errors seen on bite-wing radiographs are overlapping, collimator cutoff, and film placement.

Overlapping (Fig. 7-39, A). Overlapping results from improper horizontal beam alignment.

Remedy. The beam should be aligned in the horizontal plane so that it is at right angles to the film packet.

Collimator cutoff (cone cutting) (Fig. 7-39, B). Collimator cutoff is failure to align the central ray with the center of the film packet. It occurs most often because the operator loses sight of the bite tab when the patient closes the mouth.

Remedy. The bite tab should be kept visible by asking the patient to smile while biting. If this is not possible, the tab can be touched with one hand while aligning the beam with the other. The central ray is directed at the tab. A localizing ring can also be used to help center the x-ray beam.

Fig. 7-39. A, Overlapped bite-wing; **B,** Collimator cutoff on bite-wing; **C,** Improper film placement.

Poor film placement (Fig. 7-39, C). Poor film placement occurs in bite-wing films when either the patient is allowed to bite the film into position after the operator has let go of the tab or the patient bites in protrusive instead of centric relation, allowing the film to float free and be repositioned by the tongue.

Remedy. The operator should not let go of the film tab until the patient is biting on it in centric occlusion.

REFERENCES

1. National Center for Health Care Technology: A summary of recommendations from the technology assessment forum, J Am Dent Assoc 103:423-425, Sept 1981.
2. Sikorski PA and Taylor KW: The effectiveness of the thyroid shield in dental radiology, Oral Surg 58:225-236, 1984.
3. Bean LR: Comparison of bisecting angle and paralleling methods for intraoral radiology, J Dent Educ 33:441-445, 1969.
4. Crawford JJ: State-of-the-art, practical infection control in dentistry, J Am Dent Assoc 110:629-633, April 1985.
5. Jones GA: Intraoral x-ray film holders and infection control in US dental schools, J Dent Educ 49:656-657, 1985.
6. Council on Dental Materials, Instruments, and Equipment: Current status of sterilizing instruments, devices and methods for the dental office, J Am Dent Assoc 102:683-689, May 1981.

8

Bisecting technique, edentulous surveys

In the bisecting technique the film packet is placed as close to the tooth as possible without bending the film. Because of the anatomy of the mouth, the long axis of the tooth will not be parallel to the plane of the film with this placement. The vertical angulation of the tube head is directed so that the central ray will be perpendicular to a line that bisects the angle formed by the long axis of the tooth and the plane of the dental film (see Fig. 2-11). With this film placement, the object film distance is at a minimum. No compensation for image enlargement is necessary, and the technique usually calls for an 8-inch FFD. Although a short cone is used, this is not the determining factor in the technique.

ADVANTAGES AND DISADVANTAGES

Before listing the supposed advantages of the bisecting technique, it should again be stated that the consensus of opinion now is that the paralleling technique is the technique of choice for periapical radiography. The bisecting technique should be considered an ancillary method that can be used in special circumstances when it is not possible to parallel.

Advantages

The bisecting-angle technique is said to be easier to perform and is still used by many dentists in practice at this time. The use of the patient's finger or simple bite blocks for holding the film packets in position avoids the use of the paralleling instruments. For patients with small mouths, for children, and for patients with low palatal vaults, paralleling devices may be extremely difficult to use.

Since the film is held close to the tooth, it is possible to use an 8-inch FFD, and the objectionable, bulky, extension cylinder necessary in the paralleling technique can be avoided. This objection is not valid in the newer machines with the extended FFD within the tube head. It can also be argued that in a well-designed office there should be room for the extra 8 inches of the PID.

Shorter exposure times can be used in the bisecting technique because of the shorter FFD; hence there is less chance for patient movement. In reality, this may not be a valid objection; with the use of faster film, we are comparing exposure times of $\frac{1}{10}$ versus $\frac{4}{10}$ second (inverse square law). Previously, with the use of slower films, the possibility of movement with a 4-second exposure compared with a 1-second exposure was greater, and the advantage was clear.

Disadvantages

The major disadvantage of the bisecting technique is that the image projected on the film is dimensional distorted (see Chapter 7).

The bisecting technique is difficult to perform with the patient in a contour chair or in the supine position, as used in four-handed dentistry. In the newer dental chairs it is very hard to place the patient in the correct position so that the occlusal plane of the jaw being radiographed is parallel to the floor. All vertical angulations used in the bisecting technique are measured from this line.

Other disadvantages of the bisecting technique are related to the use of an 8-inch FFD. The 8-inch FFD when compared to the extended 16-inch FFD causes greater image enlargement and distortion (see Fig. 2-5). There is also more tissue volume exposed with an 8-inch FFD than with a 16-inch FFD (see Chapter 4).

If the patient's finger is used to support the film, as is common in this method, then the patient's finger and hand are exposed unnecessarily to primary radiation. A bite block should always be used instead of the patient's finger.

METHOD

In this periapical technique the film is held as close to the tooth as possible without bending the film. The long axis of the film will therefore not be parallel to the long axis of the tooth. An imaginary line is drawn to bisect the angle formed by the long axis of the tooth and the plane of the film. The central ray of the x-ray beam is directed perpendicular to this bisecting line; this determines the vertical angulation of the x-ray beam (see Fig. 2-11). For the maxillary teeth, positive angulation (PID pointing down) is used, and for mandibular teeth, negative angulation (PID pointing up) is used. At zero-degree angulations, the PID is parallel to the floor; this becomes the reference point from which vertical angulations are measured. Therefore it is crucial to have the occlusal plane of the jaw being radiographed positioned parallel to the floor for predetermined angulations to be valid.

THE FULL-MOUTH SERIES

Maxillary central and lateral incisors (left or right) (Fig. 8-1)

Chair position. The maxillary occlusal plane is positioned parallel to the floor, and the sagittal plane of the patient's face is perpendicular to the floor.

Film position. The film packet is held vertically so that it extends evenly ⅛ inch below the incisal edge of the incisors. The midpoint of this ⅛-inch border should be between the lateral and central incisors. The film packet is positioned as close to the lingual surface of the incisors as possible without bending it.

Fig. 8-1. Maxillary central and lateral incisors. **A,** Film packet and PID. Dot represents point of entry; **B,** Radiograph; **C,** Diagram.

Point of entry. The central ray is directed just below the midpoint of the nares, aimed at the center of the film packet.

Vertical angulation. +50 degrees.

Horizontal angulation. The central ray is perpendicular to the film packet in the horizontal plane.

If only one film is to be used for the right and left maxillary central and lateral incisors, the center of the film packet is placed between the central incisors and the central ray is directed just below the tip of the nose (Fig. 8-2).

A

B

Fig. 8-2. Right and left central and lateral incisors, **A,** Film packet and PID. Dot represents point of entry; **B,** Radiograph.

Fig. 8-3. Maxillary canine, **A,** Film packet and PID; **B,** Radiograph; **C,** Diagram.

Maxillary canines (Fig. 8-3)

Chair position. The maxillary occlusal plane is positioned parallel to the floor, and the sagittal plane of the patient's face is perpendicular to the floor.

Film position. The film packet is held vertically and extends ⅛ inch below the tip of the canine. The canine is in the center of the film packet, which is held firmly against the lingual surface of the canine.

Point of entry. The central ray is directed at the base of the lateral nasal grove, aimed at the center of the film packet.

Vertical angulation. +50 degrees.

Horizontal angulation. The central ray is perpendicular to the film packet in the horizontal plane.

Fig. 8-4. Maxillary premolars. **A,** Film packet and PID; **B,** Radiograph; **C,** Diagram.

Maxillary premolars (Fig. 8-4)

Chair position. The maxillary occlusal plane is positioned parallel to the floor, and the sagittal plane of the patient's face is perpendicular to the floor.

Film position. The film packet is held horizontally and extends ⅛ inch below the occlusal surfaces of the teeth. The second premolar is in the center of the film packet. The packet is held in position against the lingual surfaces. The operator should avoid shaping the packet to the arch.

Point of entry. The central ray is directed at the most anterior part of the cheekbone, aimed at the center of the film packet.

Vertical angulation. +40 degrees.

Horizontal angulation. The central ray is perpendicular to the film packet in the horizontal plane and is directed through the interproximal spaces.

Fig. 8-5. Maxillary molars. **A,** Film packet and PID; **B,** Radiograph; **C,** Diagram.

Maxillary molars (Fig. 8-5)

Chair position. The maxillary occlusal plane is positioned parallel to the floor, and the sagittal plane of the patient's face is perpendicular to the floor.

Film position. The film is held horizontally and extends ⅛ inch evenly below the occlusal surfaces of the teeth. The second molar is in the center of the film packet. The film packet is held against the lingual surfaces of the teeth.

Point of entry. The central ray is directed through the zygomatic arch at the center of the film. The distal curvature of the open-ended "cone" should not be distal to the outer canthus (corner) of the eye.

Vertical angulation. +30 degrees.

Horizontal angulation. The central ray is perpendicular to the film packet in the horizontal plane and is directed through the interproximal spaces.

Fig. 8-6. Mandibular incisors. **A,** Film packet and PID; **B,** Radiograph; **C,** Diagram.

BITE-WING PROJECTIONS

Mandibular incisors (Fig. 8-6)

Chair position. The patient is positioned so that when the mouth is open the mandibular occlusal plane is parallel to the floor and the sagittal plane of the patient's face is perpendicular to the floor.

Film position. The film packet is held vertically so that it extends ⅛ inch above the incisal edges of the incisors. The midpoint of this ⅛-inch border should be between the central incisors. All four lower incisors will be seen on one film. The film is held against the lingual surfaces of the incisors.

Point of entry. The central ray is directed at the depression in the face just above the chin (mental groove), aimed at the center of the film.

Vertical angulation. −20 degrees.

Horizontal angulation. The central ray is perpendicular to the film in the horizontal plane.

Mandibular canines (Fig. 8-7)

Chair position. The patient is positioned so that when the mouth is open the mandibular occlusal plane is parallel to the floor and the sagittal plane of the patient's face is perpendicular to the floor.

Film position. The film packet is held vertically and extends ⅛ inch above the tip of the canine, which is in the center of the film packet. The film packet is held against the lingual surface of the canine.

Point of entry. The central ray is directed at the root of the canine, aimed at the middle of the film packet.

Vertical angulation. −20 degrees.

Horizontal angulation. The central ray is perpendicular to the film in the horizontal plane.

Fig. 8-7. Mandibular canine, **A,** Film packet and PID; **B,** Radiograph; **C,** Diagram.

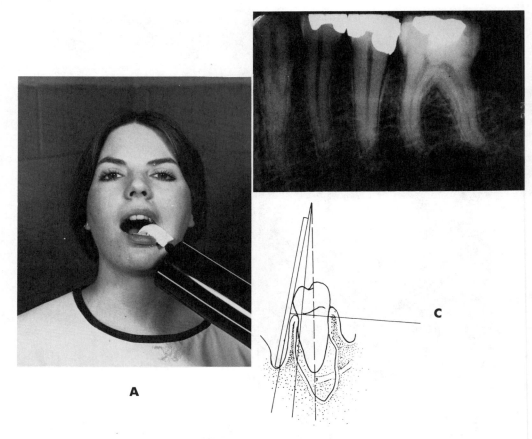

Fig. 8-8. Mandibular premolars. **A,** Film packet and PID; **B,** Radiograph; **C,** Diagram.

Mandibular premolars (Fig. 8-8)

Chair position. The patient is positioned so that when the mouth is open the mandibular occlusal plane is parallel to the floor and the sagittal plane of the patient's face is perpendicular to the floor.

Film position. The film packet is held horizontally and extends ⅛ inch above the occlusal surfaces of the teeth. The second premolar is in the center of the film. The film packet is held against the lingual surfaces of the teeth.

Point of entry. The central ray is directed at the mental foramen, aimed at the center of the film packet.

Vertical angulation. −15 degrees.

Horizontal angulation. The central ray is perpendicular to the film in the horizontal plane.

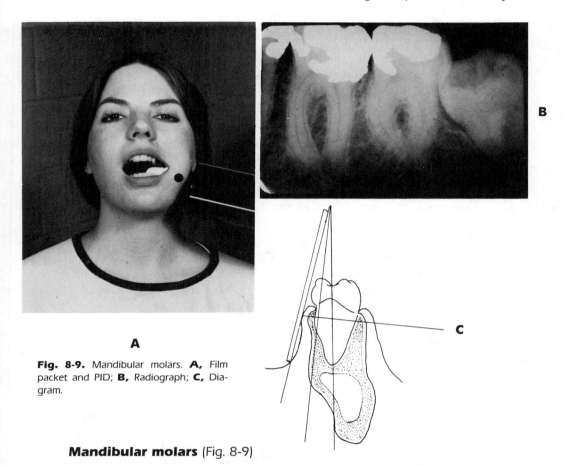

Fig. 8-9. Mandibular molars. **A,** Film packet and PID; **B,** Radiograph; **C,** Diagram.

Mandibular molars (Fig. 8-9)

Chair position. The patient is positioned so that when the mouth is open the mandibular occlusal plane is parallel to the floor and the sagittal plane of the patient's face is perpendicular to the floor.

Film position. The film packet is held horizontally and extends ⅛ inch above the occlusal surfaces of the molars. The second molar is in the middle of the film. The film is held against the lingual surface of the molars. Because of the anatomy of the area, the film packet will almost be parallel to the long axis of the tooth, and most molar periapical films done in the bisecting technique are really parallel films.

Point of entry. The central ray is directed at the roots of the molars, aimed at the center of the film packet.

Vertical angulation. −5 degrees.

Horizontal angulation. The central ray is perpendicular to the film packet in the horizontal plane.

COMMON ERRORS

The following are the most common errors seen in the bisecting technique. Recognition and correction of occasional errors in technique are important. Not all patients are cooperative or have anatomically large mouths that are easy to radiograph. It should be remembered that films retaken because of poor technique add unnecessarily to the patient's radiation burden (see Chapter 7 for a discussion of other chairside errors).

Elongation (Fig. 8-10). *Elongation,* or lengthening of the image on the film, can be caused by inadequate vertical angulation, improper occlusal plane orientation because of patient position, or poor film placement.

Remedy. The film and the central ray must be in the correct relationship. In the bisecting-angle technique the vertical angulation should be increased to correct elongation. The occlusal plane of the jaw being radiographed should be parallel to the floor. Patients tend to move after a few exposures or lift their heads to watch the operator. Their movements disorient the occlusal plane. Check the patient's head position before making each exposure.

Foreshortening (Fig. 8-11). *Foreshortening,* the shortening of the image on the film, is not as frequent an error as elongation. It can be caused by excessive vertical angulation or poor occlusal plane orientation.

Fig. 8-10. Elongated image.

Fig. 8-11. Foreshortened image.

Fig. 8-12. A, Elongated and distorted radiograph caused by poor sagittal plane orientation of patient's head; **B,** Poor sagittal plane orientation.

Remedy. In the bisecting-angle technique, the vertical angulation should be decreased to overcome errors of foreshortening.

Sagittal plane orientation (Fig. 8-12). When the periapical radiographs show the occlusal surfaces of the teeth, the patient's head has tipped away from the proper sagittal plane. This will be accompanied by elongation of the image.

Remedy. The operator should make sure the patient does not tip his or her head away from the tube head as it is brought into approximation with the skin.

Fig. 8-13. A 13-film edentulous survey.

EDENTULOUS SERIES

A full-mouth series of radiographs is taken, even though the patient may be wholly or partially edentulous. The fact there are no teeth present in an area of the mouth does not preclude the possibility of retained roots, impacted teeth, cysts, and other pathologic conditions present in the bone. The edentulous series, is usually composed of 13 periapical films. The bite-wing films are not taken, since there are no teeth to support the tabs, and only one film is used in the maxillary central, lateral, and canine area (Fig. 8-13). In small edentulous mouths an 11-film survey may suffice by using only one mandibular anterior periapical film and extending the premolar projection anteriorly to include the canine area.

The films are positioned in the same way as a regular series, but with certain modifications. The crest of the edentulous ridge replaces the occlusal plane of the teeth as the plane of orientation. The film is positioned either ⅛ inch above or below the ridge. Since there are no teeth and there may be a great deal of ridge resorption, the film will lie flatter against the palate or in the floor of the mouth, increasing the angle to be bisected. The vertical angulation will then have to be much greater. The best guideline in the edentulous series is to adjust the vertical angulation so that the central ray is almost perpendicular to the film. Any slight foreshortening that may result will not affect the diagnosis of any intrabony conditions. If the paralleling technique is used, extra cotton rolls may be necessary to support the holding device while the film is kept parallel to the edentulous ridge.

The exposure times are reduced by a factor of one fourth for the edentulous series.

Fig. 8-14. Edentulous panoramic survey.

A

B

Fig. 8-15. A, Edentulous occlusal survey of maxilla; **B,** Edentulous occlusal survey of mandible.

There are two possible alternatives to the edentulous periapical survey. The first is a panoramic survey (Fig. 8-14); the second would be the use of topographic occlusal film projections (see Chapter 9). The entire maxillary and mandibular ridge can usually be seen in their respective occlusal projections (Fig. 8-15). Both the panoramic and the occlusal are survey films, and if any suspicious areas are seen, a periapical projection of the area is done to make a definitive diagnosis.

9

Accessory radiographic techniques, other imaging systems

Dental radiography is not limited to the intraoral periapical and bitewing films that have been previously described. There are many accessory techniques, intraoral and extraoral, using different sizes of film, film screen combinations, different projections, and other types of x-ray machines as the panoramic unit. All of the accessory techniques that will be described in this chapter can be performed with the conventional dental x-ray unit in the dental office.

As with intraoral radiograph, the dental auxiliary should be knowledgeable and skilled in these accessory techniques. However, some states have laws that prohibit the dental auxiliary from performing certain extraoral techniques. Information about these restrictions is readily available from the appropriate agencies in the individual states.

Newer imaging techniques such as CT scanning and magnetic resonance imaging (MRI) are also being used by dentists to make complicated diagnoses, although this type of equipment is not found in the dental office. The dental auxiliary as an educated, aware professional should have some familiarity with these new imaging systems and therefore an overview is included in this chapter.

OCCLUSAL FILM PROJECTIONS

Occlusal film projections are used to localize objects and pathologic conditions in the buccolingual dimension and to visualize areas that would not be seen on periapical films because of the insufficient field size. The right-angle occlusal technique is used for localizing in the buccolingual dimension; the topographic occlusal technique is used for the large pathologic areas. Occlusal films are also used when proper placement of periapical films is not possible in children or handicapped patients (see Chapter 11).

Right-angle projections

In right-angle projections the central ray is directed at an angle of 90 degrees to the film. For example, this technique would be used to locate an object such as an impacted tooth in the third dimension. We have mentioned that dental radiographs picture a three-dimensional subject in a two-dimensional plane, usually vertical and horizontal. The radiographs do not indicate depth. In the example of the impacted tooth, we might know from a conventional radiograph the impaction's mesiodistal location and its vertical height from the crest of the alveolar ridge, but we would not know its depth in the bone in a buccolingual dimension. One way to determine whether an impacted mandibular molar lies buccal or lingual to the alveolar ridge is to take a radiograph from another direction. In this example it would be an occlusal radiograph, with the central ray coming from underneath the mandible, directed at a right angle to a film placed on the occlusal surface of the mandibular teeth.

Topographic projections

The angulation of the topographic projection may vary from 45 to 75 degrees, depending on the anatomic area. Since the occlusal packet is approximately four times the size of the intraoral packet, it can record areas that would not be seen on the smaller film. The extreme vertical angulations are necessary to compensate for the lack of parallelism between the object and the film. This is a modification of the bisecting-angle technique.

Film packet

The occlusal film packet (size #4) is 2½ × 3 inches and is supplied in either single or double films (Fig. 9-1), available in either film speed D or E. These films are sometimes called "sandwich films," because they are positioned

Fig. 9-1. Front and back of occlusal film packet.

in the patient's mouth with the teeth closed on the film packet, resembling the biting of a sandwich. Occlusal films are processed in the darkroom in the same way as other intraoral films.

Mandibular occlusal technique

In the mandibular occlusal technique the film packet is placed in the patient's mouth on the occlusal surfaces of the lower teeth. The back of the film packet faces the palate, with the front of the packet facing the tongue on the occlusal surfaces of the lower teeth. In patients with small mouths it will be possible to get both right and left sides of the mandible on one film if it is inserted with the longer side extending across the patient's mouth. In patients with larger mouths it may be necessary to take separate film of each half of the mandible. In this instance the longest dimension of the film packet will run antero-posteriorly. The film is placed as far posterior on the mandible as possible so that the edge of the packet touches the ascending ramus of the mandible. The patient is directed to bite gently on the film packet. For the right-angle projection, the central ray of the x-ray beam is directed from under the mandible, so that it is perpendicular to the center of the film packet (Figs. 9-2 and 9-3). For the topographic view of the mandible, the central ray is directed at a point just above the mental eminence at a vertical angulation of 65 degrees. To accomplish these angulations it is necessary for the operator to tip the headrest of the chair back and have the patient extend his or her head and neck posteriorly (Figs. 9-4 and 9-5).

Fig. 9-2. Film placement and PID position for mandibular occlusal film. Note that central ray is directed at 90 degree to center of film packet.

Fig. 9-3. Occlusal radiograph of patient's mandibular posterior area. Note buccal and lingual cortex of bone and central position of the impaction.

Fig. 9-4. Topographic mandibular occlusal projection.

Fig. 9-5. Topographic occlusal projection of mandible.

Maxillary occlusal technique

In an anterior topographic occlusal view of the maxilla, the film packet is placed in the patient's mouth with the front of the film packet facing the palate and the long dimension of the packet running across the mouth. The packet is positioned as far posterior as possible so that the posterior edge of the film packet touches the ascending ramus of the mandible. With the patient's head positioned so that the film plane is parallel to the floor, the central ray is directed at a 65-degree vertical angulation through the bridge of the nose (Figs. 9-6 and 9-7). In the right-angle occlusal view of the maxilla, the film is placed in the same position in the patient's mouth but the central ray is directed perpendicular to the center of the film packet. To do this the PID must be positioned above the head of the patient at about the hairline. The vertical angulation is 90 degrees. Since there is an increased FFD when compared with the maxillary topographic view, this projection will require a longer exposure time (Figs. 9-8 and 9-9).

The posterior topographic view can be considered a topographic view of the maxillary sinus. The film packet is positioned either on the left or the right side of the patient's mouth, from the midline, laterally with the long side run-

Fig. 9-6. Film-placement and PID position for topographic occlusal view of maxilla. Note that central ray is directed at 65 degrees to bridge of nose.

Fig. 9-7. Occlusal radiograph of the maxilla, topographic view.

Fig. 9-8. Film placement and PID position for a true occlusal view of maxilla. Note that central ray is directed at 90 degrees to film packet.

Fig. 9-9. Right-angle occlusal projection of maxilla showing palatal relationship of impacted canine.

Fig. 9-10. Posterior topographic occlusal projection.

Fig. 9-11. Topographic occlusal radiograph of maxillary sinus.

ning anteroposteriorly. The central ray is directed to a point just above the apices of the premolars at a vertical angulation of 55 degrees (Figs. 9-10 and 9-11).

EXTRAORAL PROJECTIONS

Indications

There are two main categories of indications for the use of extraoral radiographs. The first is a situation in which a patient cannot or will not open his or her mouth to allow the film packet to be placed intraorally. Handicapped patients may be unable to open their mouths for film placement, and uncooperative patients may refuse (see Chapter 11). Patients with trismus or with temporomandibular joint ankylosis will be unable to open their mouths.

The second indication is when the area being radiographed is larger than or cannot be seen on intraoral films. There are many areas of the mandible and maxilla that cannot be seen on intraoral films. The scope of dental treatment is not limited to the teeth and alveolar bone; it may be necessary to radiograph such areas as the angle and ramus of the mandible, the temporomandibular joint, maxillary sinus, or lesions that grow so large that they cannot be completely seen on periapical films.

Equipment

The equipment needed to do standard extraoral projections is minimal and not too costly. Extraoral techniques require a regular dental x-ray unit, film cassette, 8- × 10-inch or 5- × 7-inch film, intensifying screens, and cassette holders or angling boards. The use of grids is optional.

X-ray unit. Extraoral radiographs can be taken with a standard dental x-ray unit. The x-ray machine must be positioned in the operatory so that a FFD of 36 inches can be achieved. This is necessary to get a sufficiently large beam size at the patient's face. The kVp and mA of the dental x-ray machine are in the suitable range for extraoral radiography.

Cassettes. The films are contained in a carrier called a *cassette*. The cassette can be rigid or flexible and can come in varying sizes corresponding to the size of the film used (Fig. 9-12). The rigid cassette may be cardboard, metal, plastic, or a combination or these. A cassette must be light-tight and yet allow

Fig. 9-12. A, Front view of 8 x 10-inch cassette with marking letters; **B,** Cassette partially open.

the passage of x-rays to affect the x-ray film and intensifying screen contained within the cassette. The film packet wrapping in intraoral film could also be considered a cassette—a paper cassette—although it is never referred to as such.

Cassettes must be marked with lead letters to identify whether the film is of the left or right, or it will not be possible to orient the finished radiograph. Extraoral films have no raised dot to signify which side of the film should face the x-ray tube. Lead strips are also available that will imprint the patient's name and the date on the film.

Film screen combination

The imaging system used in extraoral radiography is a film screen system. The film is used in combination with intensifying screens. Previously in dentistry some extraoral projections were taken with film alone in the so called non-screen technique. Today, with the improved film quality and our concern for radiation safety, all extraoral films should be taken using intensifying screens. The screen film used is more sensitive to the light emitted by the intensifying screens than it is to radiation. The film used however has to be sensitive to the type of light emitted by the paticular screen, eg., blue light or green light.

Extraoral film is available in 5- × 7-inch or 8- × 10-inch sizes as well as the panoramic sizes, 5- × 12-inches and 6- × 12-inches.

Intensifying screens. Metal and plastic cassettes usually contain intensifying screens (Fig. 9-13). The rigid, nonflexible ones have the intensifying screens mounted on the inside of the front and back of the cassette. As the

Fig. 9-13. Cassette in open position, showing front and back intensifying screens and piece of film.

name implies, these screens intensify or increase the radiation and thus decrease the exposure time. This happens because the screens are coated with a substance that has the property of *fluorescence*. Such a substance will emit light when struck by x-radiation and is called a phosphor.

The intensifying screens produce light in the same pattern as the x-rays that have penetrated the object so that the film sandwiched inside the cassette between the intensifying screens is affected by both x-rays and the light from the intensifying screen. However, there is a loss of image detail with this intensification of the x-ray beam as the light produces a halo at the periphery of the field (Fig. 9-14) that diffuses the borders of the image and thus decreases the image sharpness.

Intensifying screens vary in their speed or exposure time requirements, just as film does. The speed of the screen depends on the type of phosphor and the size of the crystal. The larger the crystal, the faster the screen but the poorer the definition. Until a few years ago the most common type of phosphor was calcium tungstate, which produces blue light. A number of new phosphors, the rare earth elements, are now being used in intensifying screens. The rare earth elements are four times more efficient in converting x-ray energy into light than calcium tungstate crystals, and thus the screens are faster and require less exposure time. Rare earth screens must be used with a compatible film that is sensitive to the light in the green portion of the light spectrum. It is recommended that the rare earth screens with their corresponding film be used in preference to the calcium tungstate screens. The appropriate film must be used with the intensifying screen.

Fast screens are usually used for extraoral work, because the lesions we are looking for are marked by gross changes. An extraoral projection using intensifying screens would not be the procedure of choice when looking for recurrent decay or a thickened periodontal membrane.

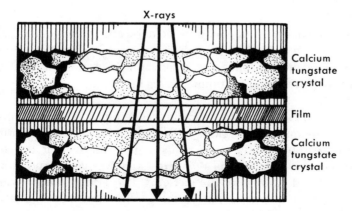

Fig. 9-14. Diagram of effect of x-rays on intensifying screens. Note halo of light produced at periphery that reduces radiographic definition.

Fig. 9-15. Cassette in wall-mounted film-holding device.

When cassettes are loaded or unloaded in the darkroom, care should be taken not to scratch the intensifying screens with sharp objects such as film racks. If an intensifying screen is badly scratched and the phosphor completely removed, a white streak will appear on the film taken with this screen. Damaged screens and cassettes should be discarded. Maintenance and monitoring of screens is part of a quality control program.

Holding devices. Extraoral film holders are available that can be wall mounted or used on a tabletop. If no device is available, the patient can hold the cassette. Holding devices have the disadvantage of standardizing techniques and preventing patient and film movement (Fig. 9-15).

Grids. The use of grids for extraoral radiography is not common in dental practice. The function of the grid is to decrease the amount of scatter radiation originating in the object (Fig. 9-16). This scatter will degrade the image by decreasing the contrast. The grid is a plate of radiotransparent and radioabsorptive strips that is placed in front of the cassette. The grid will absorb all radiation, leaving the object that is not at right angles to the film. In doing so it decreases the effect of scatter on the diagnostic image. Grids are not used in intraoral radiography because the secondary radiation does not greatly degrade the image

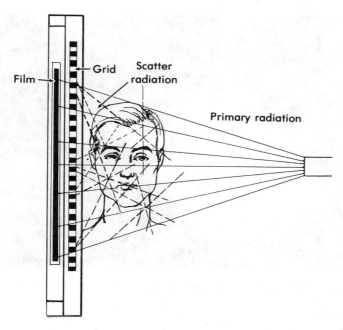

Fig. 9-16. Diagram of grid. Note absorption of scatter radiation by radioresistant strips of grid.

because of the small field size. The panoramic units, with their narrow field size, also do not need grids. Medical x-ray units will usually use grids routinely. Extraoral radiographs taken with a medical x-ray machine will have better-quality density and contrast than similar films taken with a dental x-ray unit because of the grid.

Film sensitivity and processing

Extraoral screen films are more sensitive to light than are intraoral films. Therefore what would be acceptable safelight conditions in the darkroom for processing intraoral films might fog the extraoral films. The films used in panoramic radiography are especially sensitive to excessive safelighting and may be not merely fogged but entirely ruined. Safelighting should always be checked before processing extraoral films.

Extraoral films are processed in the same manner as intraoral films either manually or by automatic processors that can accommodate large-size film. The time-temperature method is used with the same fixation and washing time as with intraoral films. The only difference is that special sizes of film hanger are used. Special care should be taken when processing the large films because they are easier to scratch when more than one film is being processed at a time (Fig. 9-17).

Fig. 9-17. Piece of 8- × 10-inch film mounted on a processing film hanger.

Projections

As in intraoral radiography, there are certain factors that must be known for every projection made: (1) the relationship of the film to the patient, (2) the relationship of the central ray of the x-ray beam to the patient and the film, (3) the FFD, (4) the point of entry of the x-ray beam, (5) the kVp, and (6) the mAs.

Suggested exposure times and mA and kVp settings are given, but these may vary, depending on the film speed and intensifying screen used as well as the size of the patient. The suggested exposure times assume the use of the rare earth intensifying screens.

Lateral oblique projection of the mandible. The lateral oblique projection of the mandible is used for surveying one side of the mandible from the distal of the canine to the angle, ramus, condyle, and coronoid process. It is not diagnostic anterior to the canine because of the superimposition caused by the anterior curve of the mandible. Before the advent of pantomography it was the most often used extraoral technique, because it is ideal for showing mandibular third molar impactions as well as other mandibular pathologic conditions.

An 8- × 10-inch or a 5- × 7-inch cassette may be used for this projection. The cassette is supported by the patient's shoulder or a holding device on the side of the mandible to be radiographed. The cassette is in contact with the cheekbone and mandible. The patient's head is inclined about 15 degrees away from the x-ray tube. The central ray is directed from under the opposite side of the mandible at right angles to the cassette. The FFD is 14 inches. An average exposure time at 65 kVp and 10 mAs would be 5 to 10 impulses (Fig. 9-18). This technique can be used with an occlusal film packet or in the reverse bite-wing (see Chapter 11).

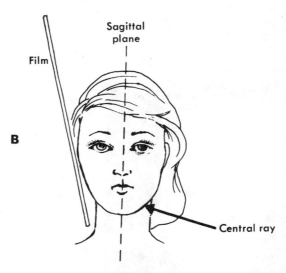

Fig. 9-18. Lateral oblique projection. **A,** Central ray is directed at cassette from beneath opposite side of mandible; **B,** Drawing; **C,** Radiograph.

Lateral skull projection. The lateral skull projection is used to survey the whole skull. The right and left sides of the skull are superimposed on each other, with the side nearer the tube magnified slightly more than the side nearer the film. It is used in dentistry to detect fractures and systemic pathologic conditions such as Paget's disease and is the projection used in lateral cephalometric measurement in orthodontics.

An 8- × 10-inch cassette is used with intensifying screens. The cassette is held in position by the patient, supported on the patient's shoulder or by some supportive device. The cassette is positioned parallel to the sagittal plane of the skull. The central ray is directed at the external auditory meatus at an FFD of 36 inches. The vertical angulation is zero degrees. An average exposure time for an adult at 65 kVp and 10 mA, would be 8 to 15 impulses (Fig. 9-19).

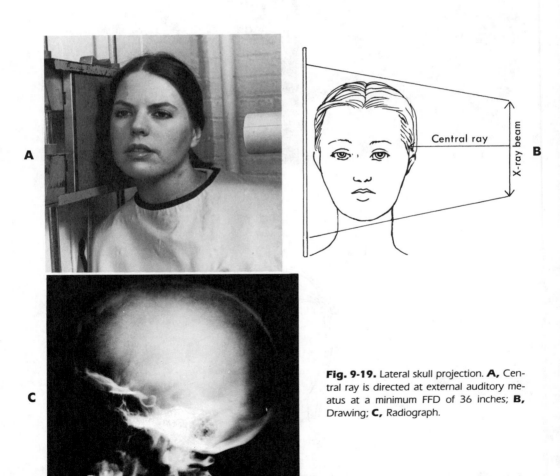

Fig. 9-19. Lateral skull projection. **A,** Central ray is directed at external auditory meatus at a minimum FFD of 36 inches; **B,** Drawing; **C,** Radiograph.

Fig. 9-20. Cephalometric unit. Note cephalostat (head holder) and extended (6-foot) focal-film distance. (Courtesy: Quint Sectograph Corp., Los Angeles, Calif.)

If the lateral skull projection is to be used for cephalometric measurement, then a head positioninig device (a cephalostat) must be used (Fig. 9-20). The cephalostat ensures that the patient's head is accurately aligned with the sagittal plane and allows for reproducibility of patient position so that films taken during and after treatment are valid for comparison.

Posteroanterior projection. The posteroanterior projection is used to survey the skull in the anteroposterior plane and provides a means of localizing changes in a mediolateral direction. The left and right sides of the facial structures are not superimposed on each other as in the lateral skull projection. In dentistry this projection is used to detect fractures and their displacements, tumors, and large areas of disease. It is not effective for studying the maxillary sinus because of the superimposition of other cranial structures on the sinuses.

An 8- × 10-inch cassette is used with intensifying screens. The cassette can be held in position by the patient, but some type of cassette-holding device is preferable. The patient is positioned with the nose and forehead touching the cassette. The central ray is directed at a zero-degree vertical angulation, aimed at the external occipital protuberance (the prominent bump near the base of the skull). The FFD is 36 inches. An average exposure time at 65 kVp and 10 mA would be 8 to 15 impulses (Fig. 9-21).

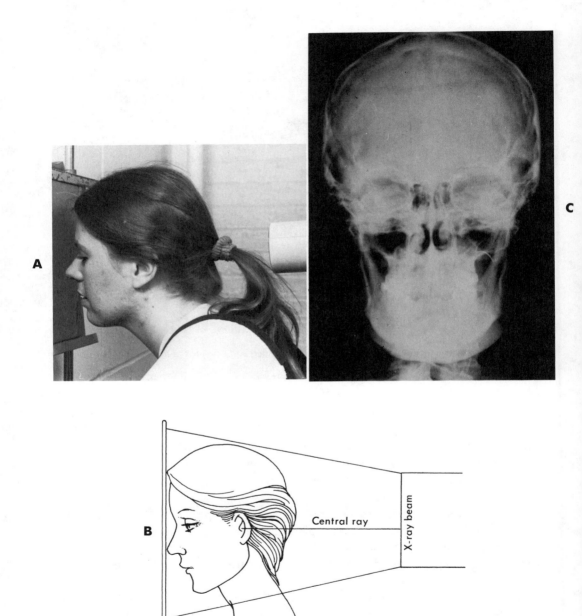

Fig. 9-21. Posteroanterior projection. **A,** Central ray directed at occipital protuberance at minimum FFD of 36 inches; **B,** Drawing, **C,** Radiograph.

Posteroanterior (Waters') view of the sinuses. Waters' view is a variation of the posteroanterior projection that enlarges the middle third of the face and is useful in the diagnosis of maxillary sinus and other pathologic conditions occurring in the middle third of the face. It differs from the posteroanterior projection positioning in that the patient's mouth is kept open while the nose and chin are touching the cassette. The central ray is again directed at the external occipital protuberance, and an FFD of 36 inches is used. An average exposure time at 65 kVp and 10 mA would be 15 to 20 impulses (Fig. 9-22).

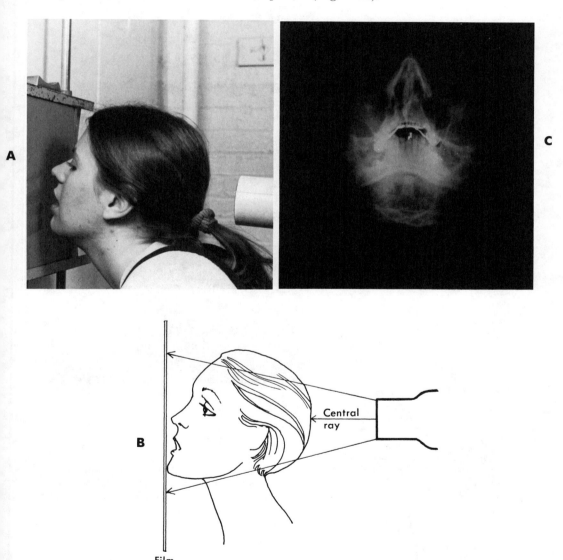

Fig. 9-22. Posteroanterior projection of the sinuses (Waters' view). **A,** Central ray is directed perpendicular to cassette at occipital protuberance using 36-inch FFD; **B,** Drawing; **C,** Radiograph.

Temporomandibular joint. The transcranial technique and modified pan-tomography are the best ways to visualize the temporomandibular joint using dental x-ray equipment. They can be used for screening when there are positive or questionable findings. Tomography, CT scanning, or MR imaging should be used for a definitive diagnosis.[1]

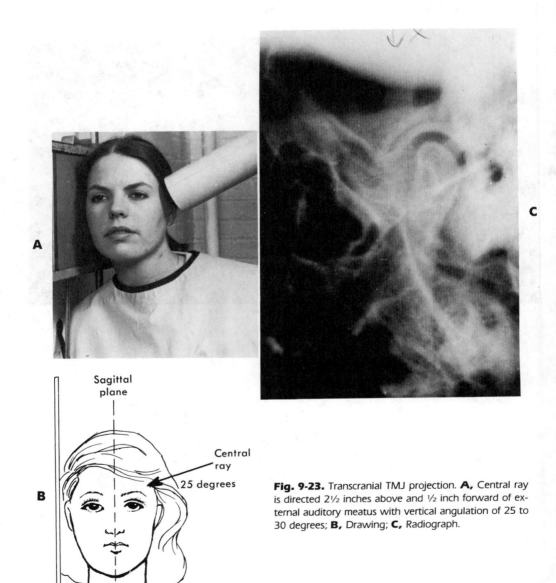

Fig. 9-23. Transcranial TMJ projection. **A,** Central ray is directed 2½ inches above and ½ inch forward of external auditory meatus with vertical angulation of 25 to 30 degrees; **B,** Drawing; **C,** Radiograph.

Transcranial projection. The temporomandibular joint (TMJ) is difficult to radiograph well because of its anatomic location. It is bordered medially by the petrous portion of the temporal bone and laterally by the zygomatic arch. Yet it is necessary to examine the condyle to look for such conditions as calcifications, ankylosis, arthritic changes, fractures, and tumors. The transcranial technique positions the cassette and the central ray so as to avoid most of the superimposition of these structures.

A 5- × 7-inch cassette can be used if only one exposure is going to be made. Usually, radiographs are taken of both the left and right condyles in both the open and closed positions. Since the diagnostic area is relatively small, the four views can be placed on an 8- × 10-inch film if appropriate lead shielding is used on the cassette. The patient's head is positioned parallel to the cassette with the side to be radiographed closest to the cassette. The cassette can be supported on the patient's shoulder or on a positioning device. The point of entry for the central ray of the x-ray beam is on the opposite side of the head from the condyle being radiographed, approximately 2½ inches above and ½ inch in front of the external auditory meatus. The x-ray beam is directed at a vertical angulation of 25 to 30 degrees. The end of the PID approximates the skin. An average exposure time at 65 kVp and 10 mA using fast film and screens would be 7 to 15 impulses (Fig. 9-23).

There are available temporomandibular joint positioning boards that are based on the transcranial technique that also incorporate means to hold the patient in a fixed position while allowing for movement of the cassette to give up to three exposures for each condyle (open, closed, and at rest) on an 8- × 10-inch film (Fig. 9-24).

Fig. 9-24. TMJ angling board. (Courtesy Margraf Dental Mfg. Inc., Jenkintown, Penn.)

Fig. 9-25. Pantomography of the temporomandibular joint. This is done using a panoramic unit with an adjustable focal trough. The focal trough is set for the position of the condyle instead of the body of the mandible.

Some panoramic units can be used to take tomograms of the TMJ (Fig. 9-25). The unit to do this must have an adjustable focal trough. The focal trough is set for the position of the condyle instead of the usual focal trough which is through the body of the mandible. By stopping the rotation and rewinding the film carrier, an open and closed view can be taken on each side with one piece of film.

XERORADIOGRAPHY

Xeroradiography was introduced to the dental market more than 10 years ago as an alternative to intraoral film packets. It was greeted at the time with great enthusiasm but has not been successful in capturing the share of the market that is neccessary for commercial viability. The unit is still available and remains an interesting alternative to film as an imaging system.

Xeroradiography is an imaging system that has been used in medical radiology for some time. The system uses the xerographic copying process to record images produced by x-rays from a standard dental x-ray machine. The system does not replace the conventional x-ray unit, it replaces film as the image receptor. Instead of conventional film, a photoreceptor plate covered with a uniform charge is used as the image receptor. The charged plate is held in a plastic cassette that is the size of either #0 or #2 film. The reusable cassette is covered with a plastic bag and is exposed intraorally in the routine manner with a dental x-ray machine. The x-rays dissipate the charge on the photoreceptor plate in a

Fig. 9-26. X-ray beam selectively penetrating the tooth and discharging the photoreceptor plate. (Courtesy: Xerox Medical Systems, Pasadena, Calif.)

pattern that corresponds to the absorption of the x-rays by the object being radiographed. A latent electrostatic image is thus formed (Fig. 9-26).

The exposed receptor plate is then placed back into the processing machine, and the latent image is transformed into a real image on opaque paper that can be viewed directly or by reflected light on a viewbox. This is done by the use of specifically charged pigmented powder. This copying process takes 20 seconds. After the photoreceptor plate is sterilized, reconditioned, and recharged, it is ready to be used again (Figs. 9-27 and 9-28).

The major advantage of intraoral xeroradiographs when compared with radiographs is better image quality.[2] This improved image quality results from the wide imaging latitude and the edge enhancement. The wide imaging latitude enable xeroradiograph to show the full range of oral structure densities from soft tissue hard in a single image.

Xeroradiographs require only a third to a half the exposure of conventional D speed film. The exposure to the patient when compared with E speed film is the same.

There is a great saving of time in producing a finished dry diagnostic image when using xeroradiography. It takes about 2 minutes from seating the patient to the produced dry image. The xeroradiograph can be viewed in direct light without the aid of a viewbox.

The major disadvantages of the system is its limitation to only #0- and #2-sized images (pediatric and adult-sized film) and the use of the rigid cassette. The rigid cassette may be difficult to place in some mouths.

The edge enhancement of the image sometimes will give false positives for recurrent decay under large metallic restorations. However, experience with these types of images will help the practitioner to recognize these false positives.

Fig. 9-27. The Xerox 110 Dental Diagnostic Imaging System. (Courtesy Xerox Medical System, Pasadena, Calif.)

Fig. 9-28. Conventional dental radiograph *(left)* and xeroradiograph *(right)* of same area. (Courtesy of Xerox Medical Systems, Pasadena, Calif.)

COMPUTED TOMOGRAPHY—CT SCANNING

CT was introduced into radiology in the mid-1970s. In contrast to conventional radiographic techniques where film and or film screen combinations are used to produce images, CT images are computer generated. CT, however, still uses ionizing radiation as the energy source.

CT scanners produce digital data measuring the extent of the x-ray trans-

Fig. 9-29. CT scan of a skull in the coronal plane. Note the gray soft tissue imaging that would not be seen on a conventional radiograph.

mission through the patient. The patient is placed in the CT unit, and the x-ray source and image detector rotate around the patient, who remains stationary (tomographic principle). Multiple tomographic images are taken of the patient. They are recorded by a radiation detector, fed into a computer, and reconstructed to form the final image, which can be seen on a viewing monitor or printed out as a film (Fig. 9-29). Although the image may have been taken in one plane (e.g., the axial plane), the computer can reconstitute the image from the stored data to produce an image in another plane such as the frontal plane. This technique was originally called the CAT scan (computerized axial tomography), but since studies are not limited to the axial plane, the more accurate name CT scan is used.

Although CT scanners are not found in dental offices, dentists are using CT in the diagnosis of tumors, pathologic conditions of the TMJ, pathology, and the planning of implant placements in the jaws.

REFERENCES

1. Griffiths RH: Report on the president's conference on the examination, diagnosis and management of temporomandibular joint patients, J Am Dent Assoc 106:75-77, Jan 1983.

2. Gratt BM and others: Imaging properties of intraoral dental xeroradiography, J Am Dent Assoc 99:805, Nov 1979.

10

Panoramic radiography

Panoramic radiography refers to a technique that will produce a radiograph that shows the patient's mandible and maxilla on one film. There are two techniques currently available to produce such films. The first of these involves the use of an intraoral x-ray source in which the x-ray tube is placed within the patient's mouth and emits a 180 degree x-ray beam that hits a film wrapped externally around the patient's jaws. This technique is not commonly used, and the radiographs produced show a great deal of distortion, but the radiation exposure is significantly decreased (Fig. 10-1). The second technique, by far the more extensively used, employs curved surface tomography.

Tomography

Tomography is a radiographic technique that allows radiographing in one plane of an object while blurring or eliminating images from structures in other planes. "Tomo" is the Greek word for section. These projections are sometimes called *laminograms,* from the word "lamina" (layer), as this is a layered radiographic technique. Tomography is used extensively in medicine and is the basis, as we have seen, for computer tomography (CT) scanning.

A tomogram is made by moving the x-ray source and the film in opposite directions in a fixed relationship through one or a series of rotation points, while the patient remains stationary (Fig. 10-2). The plane of the object that is not blurred on the radiograph is called the "plane of acceptable detail" or "focal trough." It is also called the image layer. Clinically this concept is very important, because many of the errors in technique that we will talk about later in the chapter are caused by improper patient positioning that lead to not having the desired area in the image layer. The points of rotation around which the tube head travel can be either inside or outside of the focal trough. The width or thickness of the focal trough is governed by many factors including the angle of movement of the x-ray beam, the width of the x-ray beam, and the size of the focal spot. Any object that lies in the focal plane will be seen clearly, and objects above and below it will appear blurred. By varying the focal-object distance, the distance between the tube head and the patient, on a tomographic series, different focal troughs or "cuts" can be achieved. A tomographic series is usually composed of multiple cuts, 0.5 cm apart, with the number of cuts varying according to the thickness of the object (Fig. 10-3).

Fig.10-1. Intraoral source. (Courtesy Siemans Medical Systems, Inc., Charlotte, NC.)

Fig. 10-2. Diagram illustrating principle of tomography. Note that only objects in focal trough (square) project onto the same area of the film and are not blurred out.

Fig. 10-3. Tomogram of the temporomandibular joint. Note the clarity of the condyle and the blurring of the rest of the image.

Pantomograph. A panoramic radiograph of the maxilla and the mandible produced by using tomography, is properly called a *pantomogram*. The pantomogram is a curved-surface tomogram, in contrast to the plane-surface or straight line tomogram illustrated in Fig. 10-2. In common usage the term "panoramic radiograph" is usually substituted for pantomogram. The term "panorex" should never be used as a substitute for panoramic radiograph unless the Panorex unit is being used. Panorex is not a generic term but a manufacturer's name.

There are many pantomographic units available on the market today. They differ primarily in the number and locations of the centers of rotation, whether there is a fixed or adjustable focal trough, and the type and shape of the film transport mechanism. All units use intensifying screens, with a film size of either 5 × 12 or 6 × 12 inches. Design differences include head positioning devices, bite blocks, kVp and mA range, standing or sitting patient position, and wall-mounted or freestanding units.

Individual manufacturers use trade names such as Panorex, Orthopantomograph, Panelipse, and Panoral for their own panoramic units. Each manufacturer's machine has its own technique for operation, which can be learned easily from the instructional manual (Figs. 10-4 and 10-5). With any of the pantomographic units, positioning the patient and maintaining that position during the movement of the tube head are critical. If this is not done, the desired structure to be radiographed may not be or remain in the plane of focus and will appear blurred on the radiograph.

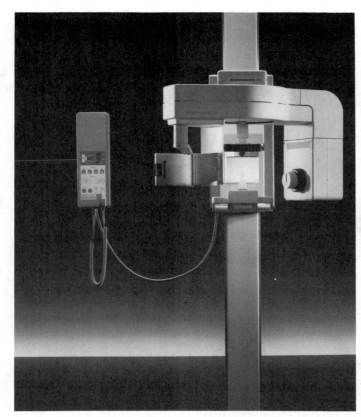

Fig. 10-4. Orthopantomograph 10E. (Courtesy of Siemans Medical Systems Inc., Charlotte, NC.)

Fig. 10-5. Panelipse panoramic x-ray system. (Courtesy, Gendex Corp., Milwaukee, WI.)

Fig. 10-6. Ghost images of the opposite sides of the mandible outlined by the arrows.

Pantomographic image. The image seen on a panoramic film will show the entire dentition and supporting bone from condyle to condyle on one film. The image-however will not have the same definition seen on an intraoral periapical or bite-wing film. This is a factor that is inherent in the pantomographic process and the use of intensifying screens. There is also a significant amount of horizontal distortion but very little vertical distortion.

All objects in the field of the x-ray beam, even those out of the plane of focus will be projected onto the film but most will not be seen. The objects that have the greatest density (e.g., bone, metal objects), will be seen on two places on the panoramic film. One of the places is the intended image or the usable image and the other is referred to as the "ghost image" (Fig. 10-6). The ghost image always has less sharpness and is seen at a point higher on the film than the desired image. The ghost image is always reversed; that is, the left appears on the right and vise versa.

Advantages and disadvantages

Like any technique, panoramic tomography has its advantages and disadvantages when compared with conventional intraoral techniques. The pantomographic unit is still very expensive, costing approximately four times as much as a regular x-ray tube head, which is still necessary even with the panoramic unit. The full-mouth series, composed of periapical and bite-wing films, has been and still is the norm for routine dental radiography, and any other technique should be judged in comparison.

Advantages
Size of the field. Field size is one of the major advantages of the pantomogram. The full-mouth series is not composed of radiographs of the entire mouth

Panelipse Radiograph and Tracing Showing Numbered Anatomical Landmarks

① Middle Cranial Fossa		⑪ Glenoid Fossa	
② Orbit		⑫ Articular Eminence	
③ Zygomatic Arch		⑬ Mandibular Condyle	
④ Palate		⑭ Vertebra	
⑤ Styloid Process		⑮ Coronoid Process	
⑥ Septa in Maxillary Sinus		⑯ Pterygoid Plates	
⑦ Maxillary Tuberosity		⑰ Maxillary Sinus	
⑧ External Oblique Line		⑱ Ear Lobe	
⑨ Angle of Mandible		⑲ Mandibular Canal	
⑩ Hyoid Bone		⑳ Mental Foramen	

Fig. 10-7. Panoramic radiograph and tracing showing numbered anatomic landmarks. (Courtesy Gendex Corp. Milwaukee, WI.)

but only of the teeth, alveolar ridges, and part of the supporting bone. The pantomogram covers an area that includes all of the mandible from condyle to condyle and the maxillary regions extending superiorly to the middle third of the orbits (Fig. 10-7). Such areas as the condyles, inferior border, angle, ascending ramus and coronoid process of the mandible, and the entire maxillary that are not visualized on intraoral surveys are seen routinely on pantomograms. Lesions that might go undetected on intraoral surveys will be detected on pantomograms.

Quality control. In maintaining quality control, good chairside technique is essential so that the undistorted complete image is seen. Full visualization of all the teeth and surrounding bone, including the third molar area, is of prime importance. This is more easily done with a pantomographic unit than an intraoral full-mouth series, because the technique, though not simple, is not as demanding as intraoral radiography. There are fewer retakes and quality control is easier to maintain.

Simplicity. Pantomographic procedures, as just mentioned, are relatively simple to perform. With a minimum amount of training and paying strict attention to detail, the dentist or dental auxiliary can become very proficient in taking these films.

Patient cooperation. Since pantomography is an extra oral procedure, it requires a minimum amount of patient cooperation when compared with intraoral techniques. No film packet is placed in the patient's mouth, and the patient is asked to bite on a rod and is only required to sit or stand still for the 12 to 22 seconds of exposure. Most units can be operated without radiation to demonstrate what the procedure will be like to an apprehensive patient. Pantomography practically eliminates problems with intractable gaggers, patients with trismus, and fearful or uncooperative children.

Time. Less time is required to do a pantomographic examination than an intraoral survey. The most skilled operator requires at least 10 to 15 minutes to do an intraoral survey; pantomograms can be taken in less than 5 minutes.

Dose. There seems to be general agreement that the radiation dose to the patient is less than or at most equal to intraoral radiography, depending on technique and how and where measurements are made.[1,2] The panoramic radiograph gives a bone marrow dose that is 20% or less than that received from a full-mouth intraoral series.[3] The panoramic dose is about equivalent to that received from four bite-wing films. This dose can be reduced even further by using rare earth intensifying screens in the panoramic cassettes. It should be noted, however, that the patient dose is relatively higher in the regions of the centers of rotation. There are also reports of significant thyroid dose during the panoramic procedure.[4,5]

Disadvantages

Image quality. Tomograms inherently show magnification, geometric distortion, and poor definition.[4] Compared with an intraoral radiograph, the pantomogram does not give comparable definition. Besides the tomographic process, other factors that tend to degrade the images as compared with intraoral films are (1) external placement of the film with resulting increased object-film distance, (2) the use of intensifying screens, and (3) faster film with large grain size.

There are many diagnostic problems in dentistry for which a high degree of radiographic definition is essential. Early detection of such conditions as interproximal caries, disruption of the lamina dura, loss of such conditions as crestal alveolar bone, and a thickened periodontal membrane all require the maximum amount of radiographic definition. Because of these factors, pantomographs have very limited value in the diagnosis of periodontal disease[4] and the detection of early periapical lesions. These are common diagnostic problems that comprise the bulk of diagnostic problems for practitioners, and the pantomographic technique is lacking in these areas. If a pantomogram is used instead of a full mouth series, it must be augmented with bite-wings and selected periapical films where indicated.

Focal trough (image layer). Areas that lie outside either in front of or behind the focal trough may be seen poorly or not at all. The focal trough or plane of acceptable detail is not as wide as either the mandible or maxilla, and only structures or changes that lie within the trough are visualized clearly. Pantomographic units that have adjustable focal troughs have far greater diagnostic capabilities than those that do not.

Overlap. Pantomographic units have a tendency to produce overlapping images, particularly in the premolar area.

Superimposition. Frequently there is superimposition of the spinal column on the anterior portion of the pantomogram. Theoretically, if the patient is positioned properly this will not happen. However, all patients are not perfect, and some have physical problems that make proper positioning difficult. The anterior teeth and periapical bone are the most difficult to interpret on pantomograms.

Distortion. The amount of vertical and horizontal distortion varies from one part of the film to another, resulting in an uneven magnification of the image; structures, spaces, and distances may appear larger than they actually are.

Overuse. This is one of the prime concerns in regard to patient exposure. The ease and convenience in obtaining the pantomograph might lead to carelessness by substitution for other projections that yield better results. The pantomogram might be taken instead of one periapical film of an area because it is easier to do.

Technique

The following are general rules of technique for preparing and positioning the patient for panoramic radiography. These rules will be valid for all units, but some slight technique changes may be necessary for individual units, depending on the manufacturer's specific instructions.

1. Explain the procedure to the patient, pointing out the importance of not moving during the procedure. Point out how the film cassette and the tube will move around the patient's head and that there is the possibility that the film cassette may touch his or her shoulder or ear gently during the exposure rotation.
2. Have the patient remove a jacket or any other bulky piece of clothing that might interfere with the movement of the cassette holder.
3. Ask the patient to remove any dentures, eyeglasses, earrings, nose rings, hearing aids, and hairpins to avoid their being seen on the film.

4. Seat or stand the patient in the most erect position possible so that the spinal column will be straight.
5. Align the patient's head so that the midsagittal plane will be perpendicular to the floor.
6. Place the patient's chin on the chin rest (if present) so that the alar tragus line will be tilted slightly down, about 5 degrees, from being parallel to the floor.
7. Drape the patient with the lead apron. Do not use a thyroid collar or a bib chain, because it will be superimposed on the image.
8. Place a cotton roll or a bite stick, if the unit has one, between the patient's upper and lower incisors.
9. Have the patient close the lips and place the tongue against the roof of the mouth. This will prevent the formation of an airspace that will be represented as a radiolucent area above the apices of the upper teeth.
10. Take any readings or measurements called for and set exposure factors.
11. Make the exposure. Since the exposure can be as long as 22 seconds as the tube and film cassette travel around the patient, it is a good idea to talk to the patient, reminding him not to move, and so on.

Processing

Panoramic films are processed with regular dental solutions either by hand or automatically, if the processor can accommodate the panoramic-size film. The time-temperature method is used with the same fixation and washing times as with intraoral films. The film used in panoramic radiography is especially sensitive to excessive safelighting and may be not merely fogged but entirely ruined. Make sure that the film screen combination used is compatible with the intensity and type of safelight being used.

One of the most common artifacts seen on panoramic films is caused by static electricity. Multiple black linear streaks resembling tree branches without leaves will appear on the radiograph (Fig.10-8). This artifact can be caused by

Fig. 10-8. Panoramic radiograph showing static marks.

pulling a piece of film quickly and forcefully out of a tightly packed full box of film or when loading or unloading film between the intensifying screens of a flexible cassette. Static electricity is produced most often on cold, dry days.

Common errors

Patient too far forward (Fig. 10-9). If the patient is positioned in front of the focal plane, then the upper and lower anterior teeth will appear blurred and narrow. The spinal column will be superimposed on the ramus and the premolars will be overlapped.

Remedy. The patient's teeth or edentulous ridges must be in the proper position in the anterior posterior plane. Check the position of the teeth on the bite block or bite stick and the position of the patient's chin on the rest. Make sure the distance setting is correct.

Patient too far back (Fig. 10-10). If the patient is positioned in back of the focal plane, then the upper and lower anterior teeth will appear blurred and widened. There will also be increased ghosting of the mandible.

Remedy. The patient's teeth or ridges must be in the proper position on the bite block or bite stick. Check the position of the chin rest and the chin for the correct distance in the posterior-anterior plane.

Patient's head tilted up (Fig. 10-11). If the patient's head is tilted up, then the forehead will be too far back and the chin too far forward. This will cause the upper incisors to be to be out of focus, and the radiopaque hard palate will be superimposed over the apices of the upper teeth. The condyles may be off the film.

Fig. 10-9. Patient positioned too far forward. Anterior teeth appear blurred and narrow. The spinal column is superimposed on the ramus and premolars are overlapped.

Fig. 10-10. Patient positioned too far back. Upper and lower anterior teeth appear blurred and widened.

Fig. 10-11. Patient's head tilted up. The hard palate (radiopaque band) is superimposed upon the apices of the upper teeth.

Remedy. The reference lines on the patient's face, the Frankfort plane or the alar tragus line, should be aligned parallel to the floor.

Patient's head tilted down (Fig. 10-12). If the patient's head is tilted down, then the chin will be back and the forehead forward. This will cause the lower incisors to be blurred. The radiopaque image of the hyoid bone will be superimposed on the anterior part of the mandible. The superior portions of the condyles may be cut off the film and the premolars will be overlapped.

Fig. 10-12. Patient's head is tilted down. The lower incisors are blurred, the image of the hyoid bone is superimposed on the mandible.

Fig. 10-13. Patient movement during exposure. Note the blurred and sharp areas.

Remedy. The reference lines on the patient's face, the Frankfort plane or the alar tragus line, should be aligned parallel to the floor.

Patient moved during exposure (Fig. 10-13). If the patient moves anytime during the exposure, then that part of the film that was being exposed at that time will appear blurred. This is different from intraoral radiography, where if the patient moves the entire film will be blurred.

Remedy. Talk to the patient during the exposure, reminding him not to move.

Large radiolucent area below the palate (Fig. 10-14). If the patient does not hold their tongue against the roof of the mouth, then an airspace will be created that will produce a black shadow on the radiograph.

Remedy. Remind the patient during the exposure to keep the tongue against the roof of the mouth.

Patient does not sit or stand erect (Fig. 10-15). If the patient slumps, either standing or sitting, then the spinal column will cause a triangular-shaped radiolucency to be superimposed on the anterior teeth.

Fig. 10-14. Tongue not against the roof of the patient's mouth. Note the large radiolucent band superimposed over the apices of the maxillary teeth.

Fig. 10-15. Patient slouching. Note superimposition of the triangular shaped radiopacity representing the spinal column.

Remedy. When positioning the patient, keep his or her spine erect. If the patient is seated, it may be necessary to place a cushion or support in the small of the back to help him to sit upright.

Failure to remove metal objects from the face, head, and mouth (Fig. 10-16). These metal objects, if not removed, will cause radiopaque ghosting on the opposite side of the film and may obscure structures making the film undiagnostic.

Remedy. Remove all dentures from the patient's mouth as you would in intraoral radiography. All objects must be removed from the face as well.

Fig. 10-16. Failure to remove metal objects from the patient's face (large earings). Note the ghosting effect of the metal.

Fig. 10-17. Placing the lead apron too high on the patient.

Fig. 10-18. Film cassette slowed because of patient contact. Note radiolucent band where the overexposure took place.

Placing the lead apron too high on the patient (Fig. 10-17). The lead apron cannot be placed on the patient above the level of the clavicles, because it will create a large radiopacity on the film.

Remedy. Keep the lead apron low on the patient and never use a thyroid collar when taking a panoramic radiograph.

Film cassette slowing down because of patient contact (Fig. 10-18). If the film cassette is slowed down or even stopped for an instant during the exposure travel around the patient, then black vertical bands will be seen on the film as a result of the localized overexposure.

Remedy. Position the patient carefully. In large-framed individuals it is advisable to run the machine first without radiation to acquaint the patient with the procedure and to check on the patient's position.

REFERENCES

1. Van Aken J and Vander Linden LW: The integral absorbed dose in conventional and panoramic complete examination, Oral Surg 22:603, Nov 1966.
2. Valachovic RW and Lurie AG: Risk-benefit considerations in pedodontic radiology, Pediatr Dent 2:128, 1980.
3. White SC and Rose TC: Absorbed bone marrow dose in certain dental radiographic techniques, J Am Dent Assoc 98:553-558, April 1979.
4. Block AJ, Goep RA and Mason EW: Thyroid radiation dose during panoramic and cephalometric dental x-ray examinations, Angle Orthod 47:17-24, Jan 1977.
5. Antoku S and others: Doses to critical organs from dental radiography, Oral Surg 41:251-260, 1976.
6. Brueggeman LA: Evaluation of a panoramic unit, Oral Surg 24:348, Sept 1967.
7. Reports of Councils and Bureaus, J Am Dent Assoc 94:147, Jan 1977.
8. Dental radiology: a summary of recommendations from the technology assessment forum, J Am Dent Assoc 103:423-425, Sept 1981.

11

Patient management and special problems

MANAGEMENT

Patient management is as important to the dental auxiliary as it is to the dentist. Besides the chairside duties, in which using patient psychology is of prime importance, the dental auxiliary will also be responsible for other patient management assignments such as scheduling appointments, handling and screening telephone calls, and collecting fees. These duties also demand the use of patient psychology to successfully manage patients.

The dental auxiliary will encounter all types of personalities in the dental office. Some patients may be very apprehensive and tense about dental treatment, whereas others may be calm and very matter-of-fact. Some will reveal their anxieties through behavioral and speech patterns; others may hide their anxieties.

Even with modern equipment, techniques, and attitudes, dentistry remains a stressful procedure for most patients. As a profession, dentistry is still plagued by the image of the unpleasant experience. This image problem is reinforced in people's minds by unfortunate representations on television and other media. There are still jokes and cartoons about dentistry that raise the level of apprehension of our patients. It is within this societal context that we must endeavor to serve our patients.

One of the important roles of the dental auxiliary—which performed successfully will make the work easier—is to try to relax the patient. The dental auxiliary may be the first member of the office staff to greet the patient in the reception area. Patients like to be recognized and greeted by name. This is especially important for new patients. It is helpful to say, "We will be with you shortly" rather than "The doctor will be with you shortly." "We" implies the team concept of treatment and stresses the importance of the dental auxiliary in the office, indicating that the auxiliary will take part in the active treatment.

In performing dental radiography, the dental auxiliary also must develop a chairside manner. Patients must be made to feel comfortable and confident about the auxiliary's ability to perform the radiographic examination.

It is almost routine in most dental offices for the auxiliary to do radiographic surveys. However, there still may be some patients who have never had dental auxiliaries perform any services for them. They are accustomed to having the dentist do all their work. These patients may be apprehensive and even object to the auxiliary's performing any service for them. This attitude should not be taken personally; it should be regarded as a lack of patient orientation to new modes of treatment. If the patient objects strenuously, the dentist should be called in to reassure the patient. The dental auxiliary should then perform the procedures.

We are striving for high clinical proficiency with efficient and confident work patterns. These objectives can be achieved through experience and critical evaluation by oneself, co-workers, and the dentist. The quality of the finished radiograph should be the same regardless of who performed the procedure. Dentist and auxiliary should be held to the same standard of quality control.

When the dental auxiliary is seating patients and draping them with the lead apron, some small talk may help to relax them. Patients want to know that you are interested in them and not just performing a mechanical procedure. This is not wasted time, because a relaxed, confident patient is much easier to work with.

Appearance is very important. The dental auxiliary should wear a clean uniform daily and be well groomed. Fingernails should be kept short to avoid trauma to patients' oral tissues. Hands should be washed, gloves put on, and the prescribed infection control procedures followed after the patient is seated in the dental chair so that the patient can take note of these procedures. If one sneezes, coughs, picks up something from the floor, or has to leave the treatment room, regloving is necessary before starting work again.

The dental auxiliary should never chew gum while working with patients. If one must smoke (and as a health professional you should not), it should be remembered that tobacco odor on the breath or hands can be very offensive to patients. Mouthwash and hand lotions should be used to mask the tobacco residue before seeing patients.

One should always explain to the patient what procedures are to be performed and how many films will be taken. Any questions the patient has should be answered if the dental auxiliary feels capable of doing so. If the question involves diagnostic judgments or treatment planning that cannot be answered with confidence, it should be referred to the doctor. Patients will often ask about the need for radiographs and the potential radiation risk. Since these questions are usually asked before work begins, a well-answered question will give the patient confidence and lessen apprehension about having the radiographs taken. It is hoped that answers to questions of this type will be found in this text, and the fears and concerns of the patient can be allayed by intelligent meaningful answers.

The "light touch" of certain dentists and dental auxiliaries is really nothing more than good technique developed with experience and respect for the oral tissues. No one is born with a "heavy hand," and thus there is no excuse for clumsy, uncomfortable intraoral radiographic technique.

Films must be placed in the patient's mouth and directions given to the patient in a manner that indicates self-confidence. A patient likes to feel that the operator is in full control of the situation at all times. If a finger-holding technique is used, when guiding the patient's finger to support the film or film holding device one should grasp the patient's hand firmly and guide it into place decisively. Instructions to the patient should be given in a firm but polite tone. Words of encouragement and praise for the patient's cooperation should be used. If a patient is not following instructions, for example, raising the head and altering occlusal plane orientation, the patient should be corrected. One should not accept improper patient position because of feeling reticent about reminding patients about their movements.

Every patient is different, both in the anatomic configuration of the mouth and in psychologic makeup. This is the challenge of the profession: to be able to perform one's duties and to maintain standards of excellence although the clinical situation may change. Through study, practice, and self-evaluation, these goals can be met.

SPECIAL PROBLEMS

Gagging

Of all the problems one may encounter in intraoral radiography, gagging is probably the most troublesome. Gagging, more properly called the *gag reflex*, is a body defense mechanism. The coughing and retching produced in the gag reflex are meant to expel any foreign body from the throat and thus protect the airway from obstruction. An anesthesiologist never leaves a patient after surgery with a general anesthetic until the patient is awake and the gag reflex restored. At this point the patient can expel any mucus or other material that might obstruct the air passage because of the action of the gag reflex. All patients have gag reflexes; some are more active than others. The areas that are most sensitive to stimuli producing the gag reflex are the palate, base of the tongue, and the posterior wall of the pharynx. It is in the maxillary molar area that gagging will occur most frequently. The level of excitation of these reflexes varies from person to person. It is the patient with the low threshold for stimulation of the gag reflex who presents the problem in intraoral radiography.

There are very few patients, probably less than 0.1%, whose gag reflex is so active that intraoral radiography is impossible. With this in mind, how do we deal with the remaining 99.9%? The following are a set of generally accepted suggestions and techniques that should be used to prevent gagging and to overcome it when it occurs. Not all techniques are applicable, nor will they succeed with every patient. One must be able to determine which technique will best suit the individual patient. Studies have shown that technique, authority, and self-confidence of the operator are major factors in preventing and suppressing gag reflexes in dental radiography.[1]

Attitude. Always give the appearance of being in control of the situation. The patient wants to believe that the operator is so competent that it would be impossible for the film to slip and lodge in the throat. Firm positioning of the film holder, with decisive instructions to the patient, and proper body language are all necessary.

Think positively; never mention the possibility of gagging. The worst thing you can say to a patient is, "This won't make you gag." The patient may never have thought of gagging until reminded of the possibility.

Film order and technique. When taking a full-mouth radiographic survey, start in the maxilla, taking the anterior films first and working posteriorly. The film placement in the maxillary molar area is the one most likely to excite the gag reflex. Once the reflex is excited, the patient may continue to gag even on anterior films.

When placing the film in the patient's mouth for maxillary molars and pre-molars, do not slide the film along the palate. Place the film in the desired position on the lingual surface of the teeth, and then with one decisive motion bring the film into contact with the palate.

Always set the exposure timing dial for the desired exposure before you place the film in the patient's mouth. Have the tube on the side of the patient's face that is to be radiographed, with the PID at the approximate vertical angulation. The object is to minimize the amount of time the film packet has to remain in the patient's mouth. Preparations like these can save valuable seconds and lessen the likelihood of the patient's gagging. Generally, the longer the film stays in the mouth, the more likelihood of gagging.

Deep breathing. It is often helpful to instruct the patient to take deep breaths through his or her nose while the film packet is being placed in a gag-sensitive area such as the palate. Why this works is debatable, but it may be that breathing through the nose avoids the rush of air across the sensitive tissues of the palate. Another explanation is that it gives the patient something to do and may distract him from thinking about gagging. Use a firm tone of voice when instructing the patient to take these deep breaths. The operator may also take some audible deep breaths to encourage the patient to do likewise.

Bite blocks and film-holding devices. Any film-holding device that requires the patient to bite and maintain pressure may also be helpful in avoiding gagging. Again, the patient is given something positive to do. Another tactile sensation, that of biting and the pressure of the bite block against the teeth, may distract the patient from thoughts of gagging.

Lozenges, gargles, and sprays. All of these may be of some help in certain situations. It is most important that the patient be made to believe that the medication will have an effect. There have been instances in which a vitamin pill was given to a patient as an "antigag pill." The patient was told in advance what the pill would do, and the rate of success was very high. This placebo effect is seen also in many other areas of dental practice. Note, however, that the patient was told what the effect of the placebo medication would be.

There are many viscous topical anesthetics available for rinsing the mouth, gargling, or spraying the palate to produce a numbing sensation, intended to block the gag reflex.

An undiluted mouthwash may also have some anesthetic effects on the palate. Many cough lozenges contain some local anesthetic; having the patient suck on a lozenge before radiography may be helpful.

In all these cases it may not be so much the anesthetic vehicle used as the manner of presentation to the patient that produces the desired results.

Hypnosis. Although the practice of hypnosis is out of the province of the dental auxiliary, its use in dentistry should be mentioned. In intractable gaggers hypnosis by trained, competent practitioners may be necessary to permit intraoral radiography.

It should be pointed out that convincing a patient that something (like gagging) may not occur can be considered a form of hypnosis. An application of this principle is to tell the gagging patient that you are going to press the antigag nerve located in his neck. We know that there is no antigag nerve, but the patient may not. If the area in the neck is pressed hard, some sensation will occur and the patient may become convinced that gagging will not occur.

Salt. One of the more amusing techniques described in the literature to stop gagging is to place ordinary table salt on the tip of the tongue of the gagging patient. The salt is placed in the palm of the patient's hand and he or she is asked to touch the tip of the tongue to the salt and then raise the tongue to touch the palate. It may be a method worth trying at least once in one's professional career.

For the intractable gagger, where all else fails, one must then resort to accessory techniques. Panoramic films, previously discussed, since there is extraoral film placement, have the advantage of circumventing the gag reflex.

Localization

Standard intraoral periapical and bite-wing films show the teeth and bone in only two dimensions—the superoinferior and anteroposterior plane. There are, however, many clinical situations when it is necessary for a proper radiographic diagnosis to establish the position of structures in the buccolingual plane. Clinical examples would include localization of impactions, foreign bodies, and areas of pathology, as well as differentiating buccal and palatal roots in endodontic procedures (Figs. 11-1 and 11-2). This information is essential to the dentist before any treatment can be instituted.

Fig. 11-1. Impacted maxillary canine. Is the tooth positioned buccally or palatally to the alveolar ridge?

Fig. 11-2. Maxillary first bicuspid with endodontic filling. Which canal is buccal, and which is palatal?

Fig. 11-3. Localization by definition. Is the impacted supernumerary tooth more clearly defined than the rest of the teeth? If not, it is probably positioned buccally.

The four techniques that can be used for localization are (1) definition evaluation, (2) tube shift, (3) right-angle technique, and (4) pantomography.

Definition evaluation. Structures that lie closer to the x-ray film will have better radiographic definition than those that are farther from the film. This is true for both intraoral and extraoral films. It is sometimes possible, depending on the quality of the radiograph, to determine the relative position of superimposed structures by determining which has better radiographic definition. Because intraoral film is positioned lingually in the patient's mouth, the superimposed structure that is more sharply defined will be positioned lingually in relation to the other structures (Fig. 11-3). An advantage of this technique, when compared with the others that follow, is that it requires no further x-ray exposures of the patient. It is, however, the least reliable of the techniques mentioned.

Tube shift. The tube shift method uses what is referred to as Clark's rule or the *buccal object rule*. Its advantage to the practitioner is that it can be accomplished by using standard periapical technique. To determine the relative buccolingual relationship between two structures that appear radiographically superimposed, a second radiograph is taken. All factors remain the same for the second exposure, except the tube is shifted about 20 degrees either mesially or distally. The point of entry, film position, and vertical angulation remain the same as in the previous film. When the two radiographs are compared, the buccal object will appear to have moved in the opposite direction from the tube shift when compared to other structures on the radiograph (Figs. 11-4 and 11-5). If the tube is shifted mesially by changing the horizontal angulation, the buccal object will appear to have moved distally. Conversely, a distal shift will result in

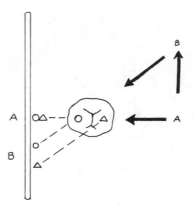

Fig. 11-4. Buccal-object rule. As the tube position is shifted mesially (position B), the buccal object is seen to move relatively in the opposite direction, distally.

Fig. 11-5. Radiographs illustrating the buccal-object rule. The tube in **B** was shifted to the mesial, indicating that the short endodontic point is in the mesiobuccal canal.

the more buccal object moving mesially. This can be demonstrated on your fingers. Hold your hand so that the second and third fingers are superimposed when you are sighting them from the side. Move your head either to the left or to the right (mesially or distally) and imagine the images of the fingers being recorded on the film. You now can see two distinct fingers and not the fingers superimposed. Now apply the buccal object rule. The key phrase is "same lingual, opposite buccal"—the acronym is SLOB.

Right-angle technique. The right-angle technique uses two projections taken at right angles to each other—first a periapical film and then an occlusal film of the same area, for example. The planes radiographed are at right angles to each other. The occlusal techniques and examples are discussed in Chapter 9.

Pantomography. The redundant images produced in the anterior region by some older-model pantomographic units, such as the Panorex, can be used to localize objects in repeated areas. In viewing the film, the object in question will be seen twice, once on each half of the film. A recommended technique is to compare the relative movement of the object with adjacent structures from one side of the film to the other with the direction that the clinician reads the film (for example, left to right).[2] The object will seem to have moved in the same direction as the clinician's viewing movement if it is lingually positioned and in the opposite direction if it is on the buccal side (Fig. 11-6).

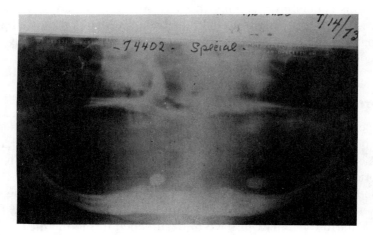

Fig. 11-6. Localization of an object by pantomographic redundant image.

Third molars

The third molars are in an area of the mouth difficult to radiograph. In many cases it may not be possible to position the film packet intraorally to visualize these areas adequately on radiographs. This is especially true if the teeth are impacted. In these cases it may be necessary to utilize the extraoral and panoramic techniques described in Chapters 9 and 10. It should be emphasized that the third molar area must be seen to make a complete diagnosis. If it cannot be seen by periapical films, other methods must be used.

Maxilla. As the film is placed more and more distally toward the patient's throat, the likelihood of exciting the gag reflex increases. It may be helpful to hold the film packet with a hemostat so as to maintain a minimum of contact with the palate. The film packet should be kept as parallel to the palatal vault as possible. To avoid distortion the vertical angulation will have to be increased, with the resulting relationship of the central ray to the film packet looking very much like an occlusal projection.

Mandible. The most common difficulty in radiographing lower third molars is the inability to place the film packet distal enough to record the image of the whole tooth and root structure. This placement is prevented by the muscles of the floor of the mouth and tongue. To overcome this problem the tongue can be deflected to the opposite side of the mouth by the operator's finger or a mouth mirror. The floor of the mouth is gently depressed, almost massaged, to relax the mylohyoid muscle. While this is being done, the film packet is slid along the lingual surface of the mandible as far distally as possible. In certain horizontal impactions of the mandible it may be necessary to distort the image in the horizontal plane in order to visualize the entire tooth with intraoral radiography. This is done by changing the horizontal angulation of the x-ray beam so that it is not at right angles to the film packet, which is the usual procedure, but so that the beam comes from the distal side and the central ray makes an acute angle with the film.

Narrow arch

In some mouths it may be impossible to place anterior film packets properly without excessive bending, with resultant distortion of the radiographic image. The best way to overcome this problem is to vary the film size. The #1 narrow anterior film is recommended, although it may be possible to use #0. There is no rule that you cannot use different-sized intraoral packets in the same full-mouth series. The only possible problem will be in mounting the films. The smaller or narrower films will have to be attached to the mount by cellophane tape or staples so they do not slip from the window in the mount. Pedodontic or narrow film may be used as the situation dictates (Fig. 11-7).

If radiographs show overlapping of teeth, especially in the anterior region,

Fig. 11-7. Periapical radiographs of lower anterior region using narrow anterior (#1) film seen on left and pedodontic size (#0) film seen on right.

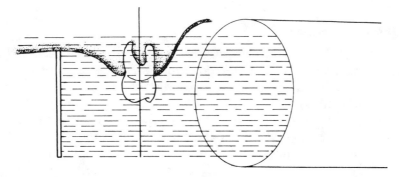

Fig. 11-8. Problem of film placement in paralleling technique with patients with low palatal vaults. Note that film cannot be placed high enough to record image of root apices.

it does not necessarily indicate that the films were taken improperly. If the teeth are overlapped in the mouth, they will appear overlapped radiographically.

Shallow palate

The shallow palatal vault presents the greatest problem in the paralleling technique. Because of the bony structures it may be impossible to place the film packet parallel to the long axis of the tooth and yet be high enough to record the radiographic image (Fig. 11-8). This technique may have to be abandoned for these patients and the bisecting-angle technique used instead. Before changing techniques one should always check to see that the film is in the midline where there is the greatest palatal height. The number of times that the paralleling technique cannot be used is quite small.

In the bisecting-angle technique the shallow palate is compensated for by increasing the vertical angulation. As long as the film packet is in the patient's

Fig. 11-9. How to overcome the problem of a low palatal vault in bisecting-angle technique. Note increase in vertical angulation.

mouth so that there is a 3-mm border projecting beneath the incisal or occlusal edge of the teeth and the central ray bisects the angle formed between film packet and the long axis of the tooth, the shallow palate will be compensated for (Fig. 11-9).

Lingual frenulum

It is extremely difficult to radiograph patients who have a large, tight, lingual frenulum, attached close to the tip of the tongue. These patients are sometimes referred to as "tongue-tied" because they cannot protrude their tongues very far out of their mouths.

The paralleling technique is not the method of choice for these patients because the tight frenulum will not allow placement of the film packet deep in the floor of the mouth. Relaxing the muscle as recommended for the mylohyoid will still not produce enough room. It is best to use the bisecting technique. Since the film cannot be placed very deep in the mouth, negative vertical angulations in the range of minus 40 degrees to minus 60 degrees can be expected.

Tori

The maxillary torus (torus palatinus), if present, usually causes no problems in periapical radiography. It is located posteriorly in the midline of the palate and does not hinder film placement. The best way to radiograph a torus palatinus is by use of an occlusal projection.

The mandibular tori, or torus as the case may be, are located on the lingual aspect of the mandible in the premolar area. Their presence prevents the placement of the film packet in its usual position. This difficulty is more accentuated in the bisecting-angle technique than in the paralleling technique. The film packet cannot be depressed into the floor of the mouth while being kept close to the lingual surface of the teeth. The only possible solution is to place the film over the torus. This increases the angle between the film packet and the long axis of the tooth and is compensated for by increasing the vertical angulation to bisect the angle. In the paralleling method with its increased object-film distances, the film is positioned behind the tori.

Canine overlap

Overlapping the image of the mesial portion of the maxillary first premolar with the image of the distal surface of the canine is a common problem. The overlapping is caused by the large palatal cusp of the first premolar. The problem can be solved by changing the horizontal angulation so that the central ray comes more from the distal side, as in a premolar periapical projection (Fig. 11-10); then the palatal cusp will not be superimposed. Overlapping does not occur in the mandible, because the first premolar has a very small lingual cusp.

Fig. 11-10. A, Diagram of changing horizontal angulation to avoid distal overlap of maxillary canine; **B,** Overlapped canine; **C,** Overlapping eliminated.

Trismus

Trismus is the condition with which a patient is unable to open his mouth. It may be partial or complete and is usually caused by infection or trauma. To make an adequate diagnosis and identify the infected tooth or area, radiographs are necessary. If the patient's mouth cannot be opened at all, extraoral or panoramic films will be necessary. If there is partial opening, it may be possible to place an intraoral film by modifying the usual technique. A hemostat is used to hold the film packet, since it is much narrower than a finger or any other film-holding device. The film packet is placed in the mouth by sliding it between the partially opened anterior teeth in the horizontal plane. Once beyond the teeth, the film can be turned to its proper vertical orientation. If possible, the patient then holds the hemostat with the film packet attached to it in position while the exposure is made.

Handicapped patients

The problems of treating the handicapped patient in the dental office vary according to the degree of disability. With patients confined to wheelchairs, it may be easier to radiograph them in the wheelchair than to transfer them to the dental chair. This presents no problem as long as the x-ray machine and patient can be maneuvered into the proper relationship. Panoramic and extraoral projections are useful in this type of patient.

The patient who has no digital control cannot hold film packets in place, so a bite block or other film-holding device is used.

It is the spastic patient with uncontrollable movements who presents the greatest problem. It may be necessary for someone, usually a parent or friend, to hold the patient's head steady while the radiograph is being taken. This person can wear lead gloves and a lead apron for radiation protection. It should not be the dental auxiliary or the dentist who constantly works with radiation, holding the patient and standing in the direct x-ray beam.

For a totally unmanageable patient, radiographs may have to be taken with the patient under general anesthesia. These films are usually developed immediately and the necessary dental procedures performed while the patient is still anesthetized.

Bedridden patients

There may be patients in hospitals and nursing homes who cannot be brought to the dental suites and for whom dental procedures and radiographs must be done at the bedside. Mobile dental x-ray units can be brought to the bed and radiographs taken. For the patient in the supine position, it is easier to use a film-holding device with a localizing ring. In treating a patient at home or at a site that does not have a dental x-ray unit, there are portable x-ray units

Fig. 11-11. Siemens Portaray transportable x-ray examination unit. (Courtesy Siemens Medical Systems Inc., Charlotte, NC.)

that can be adapted for dental use and assembled on site (Fig. 11-11). A small, portable, rapid processing tank should also be brought along so that the radiographs can be processed and the patient treated at the same visit.

Children

In dental radiography the complete cooperation of the patient is necessary. If the patient moves, the radiographic image will be blurred and the film rendered useless. In no other area of dentistry is this absolute cooperation so necessary. If a child moves during an operative dentistry procedure, it can be compensated for. In radiography the patient must hold still while the exposure is being made.

The unknown is a frightening thing to any child, and very few children know anything about x-rays. In fact, the dental radiograph may be their first in-

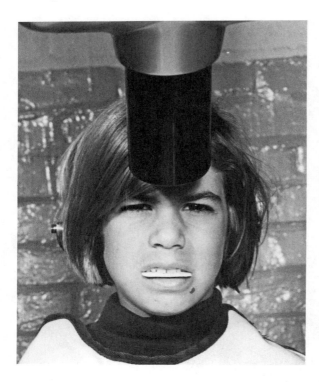

Fig. 11-12. Technique for periapical films that allows child to bite on film. Note increase in vertical angulation.

troduction to any radiography. The procedure then must be explained to the child in terms the child can understand. One should talk of taking a "picture" of the tooth with a "camera." Remind children that they must hold still when the picture is being taken. Show children the film packet and let them put it in their mouths. Taking a picture of the child's thumb is a good way to introduce the concept of holding still and to assure the child that he or she will feel nothing when the tooth is radiographed. Of course, the x-ray machine is off when these thumb exposures are made.

Children like to see pictures, and it is sometimes helpful to show the child what a radiograph of a tooth looks like. This is followed by the promise of showing the child what his teeth will look like on the finished radiograph. We have, in certain instances, even taken children into the darkroom and let them help process the films. Children are fascinated by the darkroom with its tanks and chemicals. Any effort expended to relax the child and make him or her feel at ease will reap benefits at later appointments.

Children usually tolerate periapical films and can hold them in place with the thumb or bite block. If there is resistance to holding the film, have the child bite on the film and then increase the vertical angulation to bisect the angle so it appears that you are almost taking an occlusal projection (Fig. 11-12). This type of film is not as desirable as the regular technique, but it is better than no film at all. This method will work for any area of the child's mouth, and a full-mouth series can be taken this way if necessary. Either adult-size or occlusal film can be used for this technique (Fig. 11-13).

Fig. 11-13. Radiographs taken by having the child bite the film packet. **A,** Adult-size periapical film packet. (Note odontoma blocking tooth eruption.) **B,** Occlusal film.

Fig. 11-14. Film placement for reverse bite-wing radiograph.

Reverse bite-wings. Some children will not tolerate the placement of the bite-wing film. When instructed to close on the tab, they push the lower part of the film out of the floor of the mouth with their tongue and then close their teeth on the film. If after repeated attempts proper placement meets with failure, a reverse bite-wing technique can be substituted. In this method, the film packet is placed on the cheek side of the teeth in the buccal sulcus (Fig. 11-14). The child bites on the tab to hold the film packet in place. The x-ray beam is directed extraorally from under the opposite side of the mandible as in a lateral oblique projection (Fig. 11-15). The exposure time must be increased by a factor of 4 or 5 because of the increased FFD. The resulting film will not have the detail of an intraoral bite-wing radiograph but will be a useful substitute (Fig. 11-16).

If intraoral film placement is not possible for the child, an extraoral film

Fig. 11-15. Tube position for reverse bite-wing radiograph. Note that central ray is directed from underneath mandible of opposite side while being aimed at bite-wing film.

Fig. 11-16. Reverse bite-wing radiograph.

can be substituted. The view that is most diagnostic is a slight variation of the lateral oblique technique. The cassette is positioned in the usual way, but the central ray is directed from behind the angle of the mandible on the opposite side (Fig. 11-17). Again the radiograph is not as diagnostic as an intraoral film but better than none (Fig. 11-18).

If there is no extraoral cassette in the office, a piece of occlusal film can be

Fig. 11-17. Lateral oblique technique for caries and pathology detection in children. Note that central ray is aimed from behind angle of mandible on opposite side.

Fig. 11-18. Radiograph taken by lateral oblique technique.

Fig. 11-19. Occlusal film packet used as extraoral film.

Fig. 11-20. Radiograph made by using occlusal film packet extraorally.

substituted (Fig. 11-19) but with the resulting increase of radiation exposure to the patient. An exposure time of nearly 2 seconds will be necessary because of the increased FFD. The radiograph produced will be of some diagnostic value (Fig. 11-20).

Endodontic radiographs

In patients undergoing endodontic treatment it is necessary to take working and measurement films while the rubber dam is in place. The bisecting method can be used with the patient supporting the film packet under the rub-

Fig. 11-21. Radiograph with superimposition of rubber dam frame.

ber dam with a finger. It is difficult to use the paralleling method with the dam in place because of the lack of working space in the mouth and the patient's inability to bite on any film-holding device because of the rubber dam clamp and protruding endodontic files from the tooth. It is best to disengage the rubber dam frame, keeping the saliva ejector in place, and position the film packet in a hemostat or "Snap-a-Ray," parallel to the tooth and held by the patient.

Plastic rubber dam frames and saliva ejectors should be used to avoid superimposition of their images on the radiograph (Fig. 11-21). It is helpful to punch a hole in a predetermined corner of the dam so it will be easy to reorient the dam in the frame once the exposure has been made.

Rapid processing discussed in Chapter 6 minimizes working time and can be adequately diagnostic in endodontic working films.

Grid measurement

Intraoral measurement grids are available that superimpose thin radiopaque or radiolucent lines in the vertical and horizontal planes in 1-mm gradations. The marking grid is affixed to the front of the film packet when the exposure is made. One manufacturer makes film packets with the grid markings incorporated into the film packet. No increase in exposure is necessary with the use of the marking grid, and the films are processed in the usual manner. The measurement or marking grid should not be confused with the grid used in extraoral projections (Chapter 9) to absorb object scatter (Figs. 11-22 and 11-23).

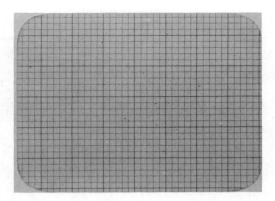

Fig. 11-22. Photograph of intraoral grid that is place on dental film packet.

Fig. 11-23. Radiograph with grid markings.

Fig. 11-24. Fistulous tract traced back from palatal opening to its origin by insertion of gutta-percha point.

Fig. 11-25. Sialograph outlining submandibular duct and gland.

Radiopaque media

The use of radiopaque media has many applications in dental practice. It is used routinely in endodontics, with the radiopaque file, to determine root length. Gutta-percha or silver points can be placed in periodontal soft tissue pockets to determine pocket depth and direction. Fistulous tracts can be traced to their origin using thin, flexible wire or gutta-percha points (Fig. 11-24).

The technique of sialography involves injecting radiopaque media into salivary ducts and glands and then visualizing these soft tissues radiographically. This method is used in diagnosing ductal and glandular obstructions, salivary stones, infections, and tumors of the major salivary glands. The contrast medium used is usually an iodine-containing formula in either an aqueous or oil suspension (Fig. 11-25).

REFERENCES

1. Sewerin I: Gagging in dental radiography, Oral Surg 58:725-728, 1984.
2. Langlais RP, Langland OE and Morris CR: Radiographic localization techniques, Dent Radiogr Photogr 52:4, 1979.

12

Film mounting and radiographic anatomy

The mounting of processed dental radiographs is another important function of the dental auxiliary. It is much easier to view and diagnose radiographs when the films are placed in mounts in their proper anatomic orientation than it is to look at them on a film hanger or sort them from an envelope. Properly mounted films make charting and examination a much more orderly procedure. The mounted films are kept with the patient's chart, and at each subsequent visit the radiographs are placed on the viewbox for the dentist to refer to.

Radiographs are identified and oriented as to position in the mouth by the tooth and bony structures visible on each film. A thorough understanding of radiographic anatomy will make mounting an interesting and challenging procedure, not one that is done automatically. Mistakes are made when there is no basic understanding, and work becomes tedious and boring.

DESCRIPTIVE TERMINOLOGY

Since we will now be dealing with the processed radiograph in mounting and interpretation, there is a need for certain terms to describe the shades of black, white, and gray that appear. With these terms we can more accurately describe the radiographic findings. The black areas on the radiographs are called *radiolucent*, and the white areas are called *radiopaque*. All structures will be either radiolucent or radiopaque, but there will be gradation in each category. For instance, metallic fillings are more radiopaque than enamel, but both are still radiopaque. Whether a structure appears radiolucent or radiopaque is determined by its object density. Thus caries will appear radiolucent, because the decay causes a lessening of density when compared with enamel and dentin.

One should never refer to a radiograph as an x-ray. One may say x-ray film, but the term *x-ray* should be used only when referring to the beam of energy that is aimed at the film packet in the patient's mouth. The film is then processed to produce a radiograph.

MOUNTS

Various types of dental film mounts are available. Mounts are made for both pedodontic and adult surveys and come with a full range of numbers of windows (Fig. 12-1). In addition to full-survey mounts, single film, double film,

Fig. 12-1. Full-mouth series mounted in **A,** clear celluloid; and **B,** opaque mounts.

Fig. 12-2. Bite-wing and single film mounts.

and bite-wing survey mounts are also available (Fig. 12-2). Film mounts are usually made of either a cardboard or a celluloid like material. The overall size and shape of the mount are made to fit the various types of viewboxes found in dental offices. The area around the film windows may be either clear or opaque. The opaque mounts are preferred because the light is concentrated behind the radiographs and viewing is easier and more diagnostic. If the number of radiographs taken does not fill the mounts, the unused windows should be covered so as not to allow the light to distract the viewer. The black opaque wrapper from the periapical film packet is ideal for this because it is the correct color and size and is easily attached to the mount.

The patient's name, the date, and the number of films taken must be recorded on each mount.

MOUNTING

Placement of the radiographs in their correct position in the mounts may seem baffling at first. However, if one develops a system based on understanding, this problem will be mastered in a short time. One must always work on a light-colored tabletop on which the radiographs can easily be seen when they are laid out. The radiographs are viewed on an illuminator or viewbox placed on or in front of the surface where the mounting is being done.

Every radiograph has an embossed or raised dot to help indicate the film orientation. The film packet is placed in the patient's mouth so that the side with the dot is always nearest the occlusal surface of the teeth. The film is positioned in the packet by the manufacturer so that the raised portion of the dot faces the x-ray machine when the exposure is made. If you mount the radiographs so that the raised portion of the dot is toward you, you are looking at the film as if you were facing the patient; the patient's left side is on your right (Figs. 12-3 and 12-4). This is called *labial mounting*. If you mount the film so that the depressed side of the dot is toward you, you are looking at the films as if you were viewing them from a position on the patient's tongue; the patient's left side is on your left. This is called *lingual mounting*. Both mounting systems are being used in dentistry today, but the trend has been to adopt labial mounting as the universal system. The American Dental Association recommends labial mounting for use by all dental offices.

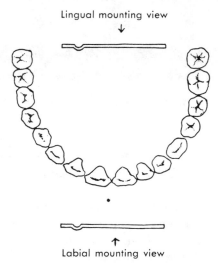

Lingual mounting view

Labial mounting view

Fig. 12-3. Raised dot on x-ray film and its orientation in film mounts for labial or lingual viewing.

A

B

Fig. 12-4. Same periapical radiograph of right mandibular molar area. **A,** Labial mounting; **B,** Lingual mounting.

PROCEDURE

The films from the patient's full-mouth series are laid out on the table top and the empty mount placed on the viewbox. The films are placed so that the dots are all one way, either up or down. The films are then divided into three groups: bite-wings, anterior periapical, and posterior periapical. The bite-wing films are easily identified because the crowns of both the upper and lower teeth are seen. The anterior and posterior periapical films are differentiated by the vertical orientation on the film for anterior teeth and the horizontal orientation for posterior teeth.

The maxillary anterior films are then differentiated from the mandibular anteriors on the basis of root and crown shape and anatomic landmarks that will be discussed later. The films are then placed in their proper position in the mount.

The same routine is repeated for the posterior films. The bite-wing films are mounted last. Since they show only the crowns of the teeth, there are no root shapes and surrounding bony landmarks to aid in anatomic identification. Once the periapical films are mounted, fillings and missing teeth can be used to help identify and orient the bite-wing films.

There are certain generalizations that can be made about crown and root shapes that are seen on radiographs. The following hints will aid the novice in mounting films:

1. Crowns of upper anterior central and lateral incisors are wider and have longer roots than those of lower central and lateral incisors. Since they are wider, the maxillary anteriors will not fit on one film as the mandibular incisors will.
2. Maxillary premolars usually have two roots; mandibular premolars have one root.
3. Mandibular first and second molars usually have two divergent curved roots with bone clearly visible between them. This is particularly true of the first molar. Maxillary molars have three roots, two buccal and one palatal. The large palatal root obscures the interradicular bone.
4. Most roots will curve distally.
5. The occlusal plane as it goes distally curves up.

These aids, along with the anatomic landmarks that will be described next will enable the dental auxiliary to properly orient radiographs in the x-ray film mount.

NORMAL RADIOGRAPHIC ANATOMY

To fully utilize and properly interpret radiographs, the dental auxiliary must be thoroughly familiar with normal radiographic anatomy. This includes all the structures seen on periapical, bite-wing, occlusal, panoramic, and extraoral projections. The first consideration in diagnosing a suspected lesion should be to differentiate it from a normal structure. This may often be difficult because there are wide variations of normal in the gross anatomy in regard to size, shape, and location that may be further modified by age, use, and disuse. Radiographically, these variations may be further exaggerated by the projection and angulation used. Not all landmarks are always demonstrated on every full-mouth survey or individual film. When confronted by a suspicious lesion, the first things considered are the anatomic landmarks normally seen in that particular area. Normal anatomy should always be ruled out first when making a differential pathologic diagnosis.

In interpreting radiographic landmarks it is important that the gross configuration of the structure be kept in mind. A thick, bony structure such as a ridge or muscle attachment will appear more radiopaque because of increased object density. Any foramen, cavity, or concavity of bone will produce an area that will be represented on the film as a radiolucency because of decreased density. Radiographs, being two-dimensional representations, will produce superimpositions of many normal structures that can be misleading, and this should be kept in mind when interpreting films.

Since radiographs are two-dimensional pictures of a three-dimensional object, they do not portray depth; teeth may be superimposed on anatomic structures in the mandible or maxilla or skull that may be millimeters in front of or in back of them. The best example of this is the roots of the maxillary molars and the maxillary sinus. Very few molar roots are actually in the sinus, although they may appear that way on almost all molar radiographs (see Fig. 12-22).

RADIOGRAPHIC TOOTH ANATOMY

The component structures of the tooth and its supporting structures are well defined on the dental radiograph because of their differences in density (Fig. 12-5).

Enamel is the densest and thus the most radiopaque of the natural tooth structures. It is seen as a radiopaque band that covers the crown of the tooth and ends in a fine edge at the cemento-enamel junction.

Dentin is the next layer of tooth structure. It is not as highly calcified as enamel and thus not as radiopaque. It comprises the major part of the tooth structure and is seen in both the crown and the root portions. On a radiograph with poor contrast it is difficult to see the border between enamel and dentin, the dentino-enamel junction.

Cementum is the thin, calcified covering on the surface of the root of the tooth. It is difficult to distinguish cementum from dentin because it is thin and

Fig. 12-5. Normal radiographic tooth anatomy: *A,* enamel; *B,* dentin; *C,* periodontal membrane; *D,* pulp chamber; *E,* cementum; *F,* lamina dura; *G,* alveolar bone.

its density is not very different from that of dentin. Cementum is best seen in the pathologic condition hypercementosis, which is an overgrowth of cementum.

The *pulp chamber* and the *pulp canal* are seen as a continuous radiolucent space in the center of the crown and root of the tooth. The fingerlike projections in the coronal portion are called pulp horns. They are seen most often in young patients, because the pulp chambers of teeth become smaller with age and in some cases may be totally obliterated by secondary dentin.

The *periodontal membrane* is seen as a radiolucent line about 0.5 mm wide between the cementum of the root of the tooth and the lamina dura. The periodontal membrane may not always be seen clearly on every root surface because of differences in horizontal angulation when the radiograph was taken.

The *lamina dura* is a radiopaque line of cortical bone that surrounds the periodontal membrane. It represents the bony wall of the tooth socket. It may not be seen on every surface because of angulation.

The *alveolar bone* is the bone that supports the tooth. It is composed of cancellous and cortical-compact bone. The cancellous bone is seen as a series of small radiolucent compartments called *medullary spaces*. These spaces are separated by a radiopaque honeycomb called *trabeculae*. The occlusal part of the alveolar bone is referred to as the *alveolar crest,* which is made of cortical bone. The mandible is a much denser bone than the maxilla; hence the medullary spaces are smaller and there is greater trabeculation in the mandible.

The *cortical bone* is seen as a dense radiopaque structure that comprises the buccal and palatal plates of the maxilla and the buccal and lingual plates, the inferior border of the mandible, the lamina dura, and the alveolar crest.

TOOTH DEVELOPMENT

The developing tooth can be seen at all stages on radiographs. The tooth germ (Fig. 12-6) before calcification appears as a round or oval radiolucency in

Fig. 12-6. Tooth germ of mandibular third molar outlined with arrows.

Fig. 12-7. Follicle of mandibular third molar.

Fig. 12-8. Dental papilla.

the body of the maxilla or mandible. As crown formation progresses, the radiolucent follicle is seen surrounding the crown of the tooth (Fig. 12-7). After the tooth erupts, the dental papilla can be seen at the forming apices (Fig. 12-8).

Radiographic examination by either the standard full-mouth series or panoramic films is essential in determining the progress and pattern of tooth eruption (Figs. 12-9 and 12-10). In this manner, conditions such as premature loss of primary teeth, anodontia, overretained teeth, ankylosis, tumors, and supernumerary teeth (discussed in the next chapters), which can affect the eruption pattern, can be identified (Figs. 12-11 and 12-12).

Fig. 12-9. Mixed dentition of child.

Fig. 12-10. Mixed dentition on panoramic film.

Fig. 12-11. Supernumerary tooth blocking eruption of first premolar.

Fig. 12-12. Tumor (odontoma) blocking eruption of maxillary canine.

RESTORATIONS

Metallic restorations such as gold inlays, crowns, foils, posts, pins, or silver amalgam are the most radiopaque areas seen on radiographs (Figs. 12-13 and 12-14). One can distinguish between them only on the basis of size and shape, not on the degree of radiopacity. The synthetic restorations used in anterior teeth (e.g., porcelain, acrylics, and composites) (Fig. 12-15) appear radiolucent and may be mistaken radiographically for caries. Manufacturers of some synthetic restorations now incorporate radiopaque particles in their preparations so that the restorations can be distinguished from caries (Fig. 12-16). Temporary or sedative fillings and cavity liners, such as zinc oxide, calcium hydroxide, zinc oxyphosphate cement, appear radiopaque since they contain some metallic elements (see Figs. 12-13 and 12-15). Porcelain jackets will appear slightly radiopaque, with the radiopaque cement being more apparent (see Fig. 12-14, A). Endodontic fillings will appear as radiopacities in the pulp and root canal chambers. Of the two types of endodontic fillings most commonly used, the silver cones will appear more radiopaque than the gutta-percha points. Compare the endodontic filling in Fig. 12-14, A, with the filling in Fig. 12-17. Other materials that can be seen are fracture wires (Fig. 12-18) and orthodontic bands and wires (Fig. 12-19).

Fig. 12-13. Fixed bridge and amalgam restoration. Note that acrylic facing of pontic does not appear on radiograph. Also note difference in radiopacities between amalgam and the cement base in the premolar.

Fig. 12-14. A, Gold post and core under porcelain jacket. **B,** Metallic pins under synthetic restoration.

Fig. 12-15. Radiolucent anterior synthetic restorations with cement bases.

Fig. 12-16. Radiopaque anterior synthetic restoration mesial of the cuspid. Mesial of the lateral incisor has radiolucent synthetic restoration.

Fig. 12-17. Silver cones used as endodontic filling material in first premolar.

Fig. 12-18. Healing mandibular fracture with intraosseous wires in place.

Fig. 12-19. Orthodontic brackets and wires.

RADIOGRAPHIC ANATOMY OF MAXILLA AND MANDIBLE

Maxilla

Maxillary incisor area (Fig. 12-20). The nasopalatine (incisive) foramen is seen as an oval radiolucency between the roots of the maxillary central incisors. In some radiographs the incisive canal can be seen leading to the foramen. The foramen is actually in the anterior portion of the palate, but superimposition makes it appear to be located between the roots of the central incisors. The position of the nasopalatine foramen on the radiograph may vary from just above the crest of the alveolar ridge to the level of the apices of the teeth because of anatomic variations and vertical angulation. In some cases, the shadow of the foramen may be superimposed on the apex of a central incisor and must be differentiated from periapical disease. This is done by taking another radiograph at a different horizontal angulation or by pulp vitality testing.

The median palatine suture is seen as a thin radiolucent line running vertically between the roots of the maxillary central incisors. It must be differentiated from a fracture line, nutrient canal, and fistulous tract.

The nasal fossa is the paired radiolucent structure that is seen superior to the apices of the incisor teeth. The fossa is also seen on the canine projection, where it may overlap or appear to adjoin the maxillary sinus. The radiopaque band that separates the left and right nasal fossa is called the median nasal septum. The septum ends inferiorly in the V-shaped radiopaque anterior nasal spine.

The radiopaque anterior nasal spine may be seen near or superimposed upon the incisive foramen. The radiopacity that is sometimes seen projecting into the fossa from its lateral wall is the inferior concha (turbinate). The concha is not calcified, so it does not appear as radiopaque as the walls of the nasal cavity.

The soft tissue and cartilaginous shadow of the tip of the nose as well as the soft tissue outline of the lip may be seen superimposed from the crest of the ridge to the crowns of the teeth. These soft tissue shadows are seen most clearly on edentulous films in which even the nares (openings) of the nose as well as the columella (separating column) are seen.

The lateral fossa is a depression in the labial plate in the lateral incisor region. It will appear as a radiolucency between the lateral incisor and canine since it represents an area of thin bone.

Fig. 12-20. Maxillary central incisor area. *A,* Nasopalatine foramen; *B,* median palatine suture; *C,* nasal fossa; *D,* median nasal septum; *E,* floor of nasal cavity; *F,* anterior nasal spine; *G,* columnella of nose; *H,* lip line; *I,* lateral fossa; *J,* inferior concha.

Fig. 12-21. Maxillary canine area. *A,* Nasal fossa; *B,* maxillary sinus; *C,* septum of bone separating maxillary sinus and nasal septum; *D,* floor of nasal cavity; *E,* shadow of the nose; *F,* nasolabial fold; *G,* floor of maxillary sinus *H,* lateral fossa.

Maxillary canine area (Fig. 12-21). In the maxillary canine region two large radiolucent areas are seen. The more mesial area is the lateral aspect of the nasal fossa and the more distal is the anterior extent of the maxillary sinus. In the edentulous film the radiopaque Y formed by the anterior and inferior border of the maxillary sinus as the arms and the floor of the nasal cavity as the stem is useful in mounting orientation.

The radiopaque soft tissue shadow of the nose may also be seen on canine area radiographs. In some projections a radiolucent area is seen distal to the canine and represents the nasolabial fold.

Fig. 12-22. Maxillary premolar area. *A,* Floor of nasal fossa; *B,* nutrient canals in sinus wall; *C,* maxillary sinus; *D,* sinus septum; *E,* buccinator shadow; *F,* extraction socket; *G,* oral antral communication; *H,* floor of maxillary sinus; *I,* zygomatic process of maxilla; *J,* zygomatic arch; *K,* pneumatization.

Maxillary premolar area (Fig. 12-22)**.** In the maxillary premolar area the radiolucent maxillary sinus may be seen either superimposed on, between, or above the apices of the teeth. It is not always visible because of vertical angulation of the x-ray beam and since the size and position of the maxillary sinus may vary from patient to patient. The floor of the maxillary sinus is seen as a radiopaque line running horizontally at its lower border. The floor of the nasal fossa may be seen as a radiopaque line running horizontally at the superior portion of the maxillary sinus. Nutrient canals may be seen in the alveolar bone as well as grooves for vessels in the walls of the maxillary sinus. Bony septum may also be seen in the maxillary sinus.

The edentulous premolar radiograph is identified by the presence of the maxillary sinus. It is differentiated from the molar radiograph by the absence of the maxillary sinus in the mesial part of the film and the start of the radiopaque zygomatic arch band at the distal portion of the film.

In some edentulous films the shadow of the buccinator muscle is seen. This shadow makes part of the normally radiolucent area below the ridge appear radiopaque because of the increased density of the muscle.

Maxillary molar area (Fig. 12-23). The maxillary sinus is a radiolucent area that is always seen on periapical projections of the maxillary molar region. The sinus may be unilocular or compartmented by bony septa. Radiopaque spurs or ridges may be seen projecting into the sinus; radiolucent tracts or grooves, representing blood vessel positions, may be seen in the walls of the sinus. The size of the maxillary sinus varies greatly because of age, morphology, and the radiographic projection as well as the vertical angulation used. The sinuses in a patient may be asymmetrical and may tend to enlarge or grow into areas of the alveolar ridge where teeth have been extracted. This process is called pneumatization. Just distal to the third molar ridge area is the maxillary tuberosity. This area of cancellous bone may also contain the posterior extension of the maxillary sinus. The large, fibrous buildup of soft tissue above the tuberosity may cause a slightly radiopaque shadow on the radiograph and is called the tuberosity pad.

The zygomatic process of the maxilla is seen as an inverted U-shaped radiopacity superimposed on the roots of the first and second molars and the maxillary sinus. The malar bone (zygoma), which is a continuation of the zygomatic process, is seen as a broad, uniform radiopaque band that extends posteriorly. Together they make up the zygomatic arch.

Fig. 12-23. Maxillary molar area. *A,* Floor of sinus; *B,* zygomatic arch; *C,* zygomatic process of maxilla; *D,* coronoid process of mandible; *E,* maxillary sinus; *F,* septum in sinus.

The hamular process is the radiopaque projection that extends downward distal to the posterior surface of the maxillary tuberosity. It is the inferior end of the medial pterygoid plate of the sphenoid bone. The radiolucent area between the tuberosity and the hamular process is referred to as the hamular notch (Fig. 12-24).

In the distal inferior portion of maxillary molar radiographs a large radiopaque structure may be seen. This is the coronoid process of the mandible. When an edentulous series is mounted, this landmark is helpful in determining which is the most distal of the maxillary radiographs.

The maxillary torus (torus palitinus) is a lobulated bony growth in the midline of the palate. When seen on a periapical radiograph, it will appear as a dense, well-demarcated, radiopaque area (Fig. 12-25).

Fig. 12-24. Posterior part of maxillary molar region. In circle are maxillary tuberosity, hamular notch, and hamular process.

Fig. 12-25. Maxillary torus.

Fig. 12-26. Mandibular incisor area. *A,* Alveolar ridge; *B,* genial tubercles; *C,* lingual foramen; *D,* nutrient canals; *E,* mental ridge; *F,* mylohyoid ridge; *G,* interior border of mandible.

Mandible

Mandibular incisor area (Fig. 12-26). In the mandibular central incisor area, just below the apices of the central incisors in the midline, there is often a somewhat circular radiopacity. This is the genial tubercle, which represents a bony growth on the lingual surface of the mandible to which the genioglossus and the geniohyoid muscles are attached. In the middle of the genial tubercle a small circular radiolucency may be seen. This is the lingual foramen, which is the exit point from the mandible for the lingual branches of the incisive vessels. Nutrient canals, although found in all areas of the mandible and maxilla, are seen most easily in this area. They appear as radiolucent lines that run vertically in the alveolar bone and terminate in small circular radiolucent nutrient foramina. The nutrient canals are pathways for blood vessels and nerves.

The mental ridge is a broad radiopaque band that represents a ridge of bone on the labial aspect of the mandible. It arises bilaterally below the apical area of the canine and incisors and runs medially and upward toward the mandibular symphysis. The ridge, if superimposed over the apices of the teeth, may hinder diagnosis. The ridge should be differentiated from the internal oblique ridge.

The shadow of the lip is seen on anterior radiographs. That portion of the film not covered by the lip will appear darker than the rest of the film because there is no soft tissue attenuation in the area. The lip line, unless identified as such, can hinder radiographic interpretation.

The inferior border of the mandible is seen as a broad radiopaque band that represents the thick cortical bone of this area.

Mandibular canine area (Fig. 12-27). The anterior extension of the internal oblique ridge and submandibular fossa can be seen in the canine area.

The edentulous mandibular canine may be difficult to orient in the mount. One should look for the genial tubercle on the mesial part of the film and possibly the mental foramen in the distal part. The edentulous alveolar ridge crest will slope downward as it goes distally.

Mandibular premolar area (Fig. 12-28). The mental foramen is seen as a round or oval radiolucency found near the apices of the premolars. The mental foramen may be found between, below, or even superimposed on the apices of the premolars. It is through this foramen that the mental nerves and blood vessels emerge. In some cases the radiolucent mandibular canal can be seen leading directly to the foramen. The mental foramen in many cases because of its superimposition on the apices of the premolar must be differentiated from periapical pathology.

The termination of the external oblique ridge can be seen in this area as well as the internal oblique ridge, submandibular fossa, and inferior border of the mandible.

Fig. 12-27. Mandibular canine area. *A,* Alveolar ridge; *B,* inferior border of mandible; *C,* internal oblique ridge; *D,* submandibular fossa; *E,* mental foramen; *F,* mental ridge; *G,* periapical pathology.

The mandibular tori (torus mandibularis), although not strictly considered normal landmarks, are included in this section because of their frequency. They are seen singularly or multiply and usually bilaterally on the lingual aspects of the mandible in or near the premolar region. They appear as clearly outlined radiopacities (Fig. 12-29).

The edentulous premolar film is identified and oriented for mounting by the presence of the mental foramen and the ending of the external oblique ridge. The crest of the edentulous alveolar ridge tends to rise as it goes mesially.

Fig. 12-28. Mandibular premolar area. *A*, Mental foramen; *B*, mandibular canal; *C*, inferior border of the mandible; *D*, submandibular fossa; *E*, internal oblique ridge; *F*, external oblique ridge.

Fig. 12-29. Mandibular tori.

Mandibular molar area (Fig. 12-30). The mandibular canal is seen as a radiolucent band below the apices of the posterior teeth, originating at the mandibular foramen and running downward and forward to end at the mental foramen. It is bordered by thin, radiopaque lines.

The oblique ridges refer to the internal and external oblique ridges. The external ridge, a continuation of the anterior border of the ramus, is seen as a radiopaque line that passes diagonally down and forward across the molar region. The internal or mylohyoid ridge is a radiopaque line that runs from the medial and anterior aspect of the ramus downward and forward to end at the lower border of the symphysis. When these two ridges are seen together, the internal oblique ridge is the lower of the two radiopaque lines.

The submandibular fossa is seen as a radiolucent area below the internal oblique (mylohyoid) ridge. It represents an area of reduced thickness of bone caused by a depression on the medial surface of the mandible. This radiolucency may be accentuated by a prominent mylohyoid ridge and a thick, opaque, inferior border of the mandible.

Nutrient canals are seen commonly in the molar region, especially when it is edentulous.

Fig. 12-30. Mandibular molar area. *a*, Mandibular canal; *b*, external oblique ridge; *c*, internal oblique ridge; *d*, submandibular fossa; *e*, inferior border of mandible.

RADIOGRAPHIC ANATOMY FOR PANORAMIC FILMS

The normal radiographic anatomy for panoramic films is seen in Fig. 12-31. Some of the anatomic landmarks listed were described in the preceding section on periapical radiographs. Those landmarks commonly seen on panoramic films that are diagnostically important are also discussed here.

Fig. 12-31. Panoramic film. *a,* Mandibular foramen; *b,* pharyngeal air space; *c,* styloid process; *d,* maxillary sinus; *e,* coronoid process; *f,* articular eminence; *g,* glenoid fossa; *h,* hard palate; *i,* mental foramen; *j,* mandibular condyle; *k,* mandibular canal; *l,* mental foramen; *m,* nasal fossa; *n,* nasal septum; *o,* cervical vertebra; *p,* zygoma; *q,* inferior turbinate; *r,* external auditory meatus; *s,* orbit.

Mandibular foramen. The mandibular foramen appears as an oval radiolucency that is seen at the origin of the mandibular canal at the midpoint of the ramus of the mandible.

Pharyngeal air space. The pharyngeal air space appears as a bilateral, symmetrical, radiolucent band that is seen between the radiopaque palatal line and the apices of the maxillary posterior teeth. It runs posteriorly and downward across the ramus and into the soft tissues of the neck. The appearance of the air space on radiographs varies depending on the position of the tongue and thus the air above it and the state of contraction of the pharyngeal muscles. The diagnostic key for the air space is the bilateral and symmetrical appearance that can be followed running distally off the bone into the soft tissue.

Styloid process. The styloid process is a radiopaque projection that may be seen bilaterally projecting downward just posterior to the ramus of the mandible. The styloid ligaments attached to the process may calcify and give the appearance of an abnormally long styloid process. The calcification of the ligament may not be continuous or may start at the attachment of the ligament to the styloid process, giving the appearance of a fracture of the styloid process (Fig. 12-32).

Mandibular condyle. The condyle, condylar neck, sigmoid notch, and coronoid process of the mandible are seen on panoramic films. Unless the unit has a variable focal plane, this is not the best way to view the condyle, because it does not lie within the usual focal trough.

Fig. 12-32. Calcified styloid ligament.

OCCLUSAL PROJECTIONS (FIGS. 12-33 AND 12-34)

It is important to keep in mind in the interpretation of occlusal films that the projection is in the superoinferior plane and shows the third dimension not seen in periapical, bite-wing, and panoramic films. The type of occlusal projection used, right-angle or topographic (65 degrees), should also be considered because the position of the landmarks will vary, depending on the angulation used.

Fig. 12-33. Maxillary occlusal film. *a,* Nasolacrimal duct; *b,* anterior palatine foramen; *c,* maxillary sinus; *d,* nasal fossa; *e,* lateral wall of nasal fossa; *f,* lateral wall of maxillary sinus.

Fig. 12-34. Mandibular occlusal film. *a,* Genial tubercles; *b,* interior border; *c,* buccal cortical plate; *d,* lingual cortical plate; *e,* shadow of tongue.

EXTRAORAL PROJECTIONS

The most commonly seen and important landmarks for the extraoral techniques described in Chapter 9 are given in Figs. 12-35 to 12-39.

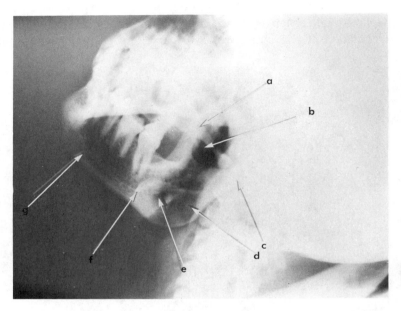

Fig. 12-35. Lateral oblique projection of mandible. *a,* Coronoid process; *b,* sigmoid notch; *c,* condyle; *d,* pharyngeal air space. *e,* mandibular foramen; *f,* mandibular canal; *g,* mental foramen.

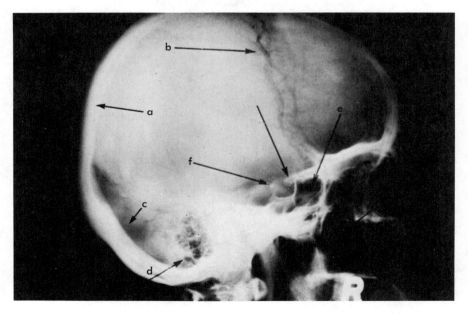

Fig. 12-36. Lateral skull projection. *a,* Inner and outer table; *b,* vascular markings; *c,* lateral venous sinus; *d,* mastoid air cells; *e,* sphenoid sinus; *f,* anterior and posterior clinoid processes, sella turcica.

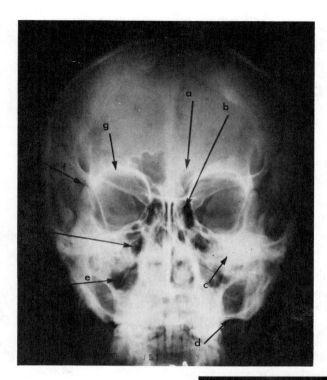

Fig. 12-37. Posteroanterior view. *a,* Frontal sinus; *b,* ethmoid sinus; *c,* petrous ridge; *d,* base of skull; *e,* maxillary sinus; *f,* frontozygomatic suture; *g,* orbit.

Fig. 12-38. Posteroanterior view of sinuses (Waters' view). *a,* Orbit; *b,* maxillary sinus; *c,* coronoid process; *d,* foramen magnum and vertebra; *e,* lateral wall of maxillary sinus; *f,* zygomatic arch; *g,* malar bone; *h,* frontozygomatic suture; *i,* ethmoid sinus; *j,* frontal sinus.

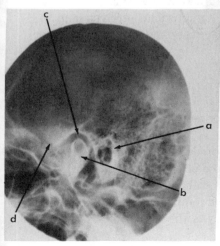

Fig. 12-39. Normal temporomandibular joint. *a,* External auditory meatus; *b,* condyle; *c,* articular fossa; *d,* articular eminence.

13

Radiographic interpretation: developmental disturbances of teeth and bone

The inclusion in this text of two chapters on interpretation is not meant to imply that it is the role of the dental auxiliary to make the final radiographic diagnosis. At the present time the final diagnostic role rests with the dentist. The importance of interpretive skills for dental auxiliaries is so that they can identify all normal anatomic structures, both tooth and bone, and artifacts visible on intraoral radiographs and pantomographs as well as identify deviation in radiographic form and density from normal structures.[1] However, to produce adequate diagnostic films the dental auxiliary must know what relevant information is being sought from the radiograph. This will make the taking of radiographs a more challenging, interesting, and rewarding process. If one knows how periapical pathologic conditions appear radiographically, one also understands the necessity of seeing the entire periapical area of the tooth in question to make a proper diagnosis. If the dental auxiliary knows how difficult or in some cases how impossible it is to interpret caries on radiographs with horizontal overlapping of the teeth, it should motivate the auxiliary to try to avoid this error in technique.

The purpose of Chapters 13 and 14 is to give the dental auxiliary some basic understanding of radiographic interpretation, to stimulate interest, and to show the importance of producing an adequate diagnostic radiograph.

ERUPTION OF TEETH

Periapical radiographs of patients up to the age of 12 will reveal some evidence of a mixed dentition. The permanent teeth or tooth buds are seen apically to the deciduous teeth they will replace (Fig. 13-1, *A* and *B*). The first and second permanent molars, which have no deciduous predecessors, can also be seen in various stages of formation (Fig. 13-2). The force of the erupting permanent tooth will cause resorption of the deciduous roots, with resulting loosening and loss of the tooth (Fig. 13-3). If root formation is not complete, a radiolucent area may appear around the root tip. This radiolucency is the dental root sack and

Fig. 13-1. A, Maxillary central incisor area in child. Permanent teeth are seen in bone. Note root resorption of deciduous central incisor due to eruptive force. **B.** Mixed dentition mandibular molar area.

Fig. 13-2. Mandibular mixed dentition. Note incomplete root formation on second premolar, second molar, and developing third molar.

A

B

Fig. 13-3. Root resorption of deciduous second molar. **A,** Early; **B,** Late.

Fig. 13-4. Root sack on developing first permanent molar.

should not be confused with periapical pathologic conditions (Fig. 13-4). There is a range of plus or minus 9 months in the normal development and eruption time of the dentition. Systemic diseases such as hypopituitarism and hypothyroidism will cause retarded development; other diseases such as cleidocranial dysostosis can cause overretention of the primary teeth and retarded permanent tooth eruption.

IMPACTED TEETH

The radiograph is the prime diagnostic tool in locating and defining the relative position of the impacted tooth because most impacted teeth are not visible on intraoral examination. The maxillary and mandibular third molars are the most common impactions. These teeth must be localized not only in their mesiodistal position by periapical, panoramic, or lateral oblique films but also in the buccolingual relationship by occlusal films.

Radiographically, the bony impaction may be seen completely or partially covered by bone (Fig. 13-5). A soft tissue impaction will not be covered by bone, but in many cases the outline of the covering soft tissue can be seen on the radiograph (Fig. 13-6).

Radiographs of impacted teeth must show the entire tooth and at least 3 to 4 mm of surrounding bone. If this cannot be done by using periapical projections, then panoramic or extraoral projections should be utilized. If the entire tooth is not seen, a lesion such as the dentigerous cyst seen in Fig. 13-7 might be missed, with the resulting disastrous consequences for the patient.

Fig. 13-5. Bony impaction ·of mandibular third molar. Note relationship of tooth to mandibular canal and root reasorption of second molar.

Fig. 13-6. Soft tissue impaction. Note supernumerary tooth in premolar area.

A

Fig. 13-7. A, Impacted mandibular third molar not seen completely. **B,** Panoramic radiograph shows extent of dentigerous cyst.

B

SUPERNUMERARY TEETH (HYPERDONTIA)

Supernumerary or extra teeth, as well as their relative position to other teeth, are easily detectable on the proper radiographs. As with impacted teeth, the buccolingual relationship can be established by the use of occlusal films. The most common supernumerary teeth are mandibular premolars, maxillary incisors, and fourth molars (Fig. 13-6) (Fig. 13-8). If the supernumerary tooth occurs between the maxillary central incisors, it is called a mesiodens (Fig. 13-9). If it is positioned distal to the third molar, it can be referred to as a distodens.

Fig. 13-8. Supernumerary premolar seen on occlusal view.

Fig. 13-9. Mesiodens. Supernumerary tooth between the central incisors.

Fig. 13-10. Supernumerary roots. After extraction it was found that there were two distal roots on the first molar. Note how wide distal root is.

Supernumerary teeth may erupt into the mouth or remain impacted. If impacted, they may delay or prevent the eruption of the normal dentition. Supernumerary roots can also occur on teeth that may or may not be detected radiographically (Fig. 13-10).

CONGENITALLY MISSING TEETH

Hypodontia is the failure of teeth to develop. It can occur in either the primary or adult dentition. It can be a single missing tooth, many missing teeth (oligodontia), or complete absence of teeth (anodontia). Missing teeth can be detected clinically. The diagnosis of hypodontia can only be definitely made by radiographic examination of the underlying bone (Fig. 13-11).

ENAMEL PEARLS

Enamel pearls (enameloma) are small spherical-shaped pieces of enamel attached to the roots of teeth. Enamel pearls are usually seen at the trifurcation of maxillary molars or the bifurcation of mandibular molars. They are asymptomatic and are usually discovered through routine radiographic examination (Fig. 13-12).

FUSION

Fusion is a condition that results from the joining of two teeth early in their development. There is usually a single large crown with two root canals (Fig. 13-13).

Fig. 13-11. Anodontia. Note absence of permanent lateral incisor and canine.

Fig. 13-12. Enamel pearl.

Fig. 13-13. Fusion. Note single crown with two root canals.

Fig. 13-14. Gemination. Note two crowns with common root canal.

GEMINATION

Gemination occurs when a single tooth germ splits during its development. It usually appears as two crowns with a common root canal (Fig. 13-14).

CONCRESCENCE

Concrescence is the joining of two or more teeth by cementum. Although seen radiographically, it may be very difficult to differentiate concrescence from teeth in close contact or those that are superimposed on one another.

DENS INVAGINATUS

Dens invaginatus, or *dens en dente,* is not a "tooth within a tooth," as it is commonly referred to, but is an invagination of the enamel organ within the body of the tooth. The point of invagination of the enamel is usually the cingulum of the tooth (Fig. 13-15).

DILACERATION

Dilaceration is a permanent distortion of the shape and relationship of either the crown or the root of the tooth. It is thought to be caused by trauma during the development of the tooth (Fig. 13-16).

Fig. 13-15. Dens invaginatus.

Fig. 13-16. Dilaceration. Note the curved root on first premolar.

MALPOSITION OF TEETH

Teeth that do not occupy their normal position in the mouth are said to be malposed. They may be prevented from achieving their normal position by tumors, cysts, supernumerary teeth, or lack of space. If a tooth occupies the normal position of another tooth, it is said to be transposed.

AMELOGENESIS IMPERFECTA

Amelogenesis imperfecta is a hereditary disturbance that affects both the primary and secondary dentition. The dentin and root formation is normal. The enamel on the teeth is thin, of poor quality, and may fracture away completely. Radiographically, the absence of enamel or thin enamel is seen (Fig. 13-17).

DENTINOGENESIS IMPERFECTA

Dentinogenesis imperfecta is also a hereditary disturbance that affects both the primary and secondary dentition. It is characterized by poor enamel that may wear thin or chip, early calcification of the pulp chambers and canals, and short roots especially noticeable in the permanent teeth (Fig. 13-18).

Fig. 13-17. Amelogenesis imperfecta.

Fig. 13-18. Dentinogenesis imperfecta.

Radiolucent versus radiopaque

In describing or in some cases categorizing bone lesions, we use the terms radiopaque, radiolucent, or mixed. A radiopaque lesion would indicate an increase in the density of the bone or new calcified material being formed (e.g., osteoma), whereas a radiolucent lesion would indicate a decrease in density or destruction of bone (e.g., cyst). The mixed lesions would have both processes occurring (e.g., cementoma).

FISSURAL CYSTS

Fissural cysts are always found in predictable anatomic locations, because they develop along embryonic suture lines. The nasopalatine cyst is seen as a radiolucency in the midline near the apices of the maxillary central incisors. The globulomaxillary cyst is always seen as a pear-shaped radiolucency between the maxillary lateral incisor and canine. The median palatine cyst is seen as an oval radiolucency in the midline of the palate. The nasopalatine and globulomaxillary cysts are seen on periapical films of their respective areas; the median palatine cyst is seen best on occlusal films (Figs. 13-19 to 13-21).

Fig. 13-19. Nasopalatine cyst.

Fig. 13-20. Globulomaxillary cyst.

Fig. 13-21. Median palatine cyst seen on occlusal film.

Fig. 13-22. Cleft palate. Note radiolucent defect between lateral incisor and canine.

CLEFT PALATE

The failure of embryonic processes to fuse in development causes clefts. These clefts can occur in the hard or soft palate or both. Clefts can disturb the dental lamina, and so anodontia, malposition, or supernumerary teeth may result. Radiographically, the cleft appears as a continuous radiolucent band (Fig. 13-22).

Fig. 13-23. Dentigerous cyst seen on lateral oblique film.

Fig. 13-24. Dentigerous cyst seen on mandibular occlusal film.

DENTIGEROUS CYST

A dentigerous cyst forms when the developing tooth bud undergoes cystic degeneration. The cyst may surround or be lateral to the developing tooth. If cystic formation begins from the dental lamina before the tooth bud forms, this is called a primordial cyst (Figs. 13-23 and 13-24).

REFERENCE

1. Curriculum guidelines for dental radiology of hygiene and dental assisting education, J Dent Educ 51:8, 1987.

14

Radiographic interpretation: caries, periodontal disease, and pulpal, periapical, and bone lesions

CARIES

Detection of caries is probably the most frequent reason for taking dental radiographs. Caries is seen on radiographs as a radiolucency in the crowns and roots of teeth. The caries process is one of demineralization of the hard tooth structure with subsequent destruction. This decrease in density allows greater penetration of the x-rays in the carious area and resultant radiolucency on the film. The degree of radiolucency on a given film will be determined by the extent of the caries in the buccolingual plane in relation to the density of the overlying tooth structure. Radiographic interpretation of caries can be misleading in regard to relative depth and position in the tooth, as well as differentiation from other radiolucencies. Caries will always be farther advanced clinically than the radiographs indicate, because the bacterial penetration of the dentinal tubules and early demineralization will not produce significant changes in density to affect the penetration pattern. The depth of the caries in relation to the pulp can also be misleading. Since the radiograph portrays a three-dimensional object in two planes, what may seem to be an obvious pulpal exposure radiographically may be the result of superimposition of images.

Caries that occurs only in the enamel is said to be incipient and is difficult to detect radiographically because there has not been any great change in the density of the tooth structure. Most advanced caries involving dentin in either the crown or the root of the tooth will be seen on properly taken radiographs. However, small, deep occlusal, buccal, or lingual carious lesions may not be seen. This is because the decrease in density caused by the caries is small compared with the total buccolingual density of the tooth.

It is in the diagnosis of interproximal decay that radiographs are most important. Interproximal caries is best seen on bite-wing radiographs (Fig.14-1). If the paralleling technique is used, caries is also seen well and undistorted on periapical films (Fig. 14-2). In the bisecting-angle technique the vertical angulation may distort or even mask interproximal caries. This is especially true of recurrent decay under old restorations. Bite-wing radiographs are also useful in detecting poor contact, fit, and contour of metallic fillings, as well as overhangs and broken fillings (see Fig. 14-1).

Fig. 14-1. A, Interproximal caries on bite-wing radiograph; *a,* recurrent; *b,* incipient; *c,* advanced; *d,* open contact; **B,** Caries seen on periapical film of maxillary incisors.

Fig. 14-2. Caries seen on periapical radiograph. Note faulty contour on restorations and periapical radiolucency.

Horizontal angulation, as mentioned in Chapter 7, is extremely important in caries diagnosis because an overlapped film will not show the interproximal surfaces clearly and therefore will be of no diagnostic value (see Figs. 7-28 and 7-29).

Occlusal caries

A careful clinical examination with a mouth mirror and an explorer will detect occlusal caries earlier than will radiographic interpretation. The absence of radiographic findings is a result of the superimposition of the dense buccal and lingual cusps on the relatively small carious area in the occlusal pits and fissures. Occlusal caries is not seen radiographically until it has reached the dentoenamel junctions, at which point it appears as a horizontal radiolucent line. As the decay progresses into the dentin, it appears as a diffuse radiolucent area with poorly defined borders. This appearance differentiates it from advanced buccal or lingual decay, which has more defined borders (Fig. 14-3). This radiographic differentiation is always confirmed clinically.

A

B

Fig. 14-3. A, Occlusal caries in mandibular first molar; **B,** Advanced occlusal caries in maxillary second molar, pulpal exposure in mandibular second molar. List the other carious lesions seen on this film.

Very often radiographs of teeth with deep or broad occlusal pits and fissures will show radiolucencies that resemble caries. These normal variants can be differentiated by examination with a mirror and an explorer.

Buccal and lingual caries

Early lesions on these surfaces may be very difficult, if not impossible, to detect radiographically because of the superimposition of the densities of normal tooth structures. As the caries progresses the radiolucency is characterized by its well-defined borders. Although it is theoretically possible to differentiate radiographically between buccal and lingual decay on the basis of sharpness of the image, it is not clinically important. The differentiation is done more easily with a mirror and an explorer. It is impossible to judge the relationship of buccal or lingual caries to the pulp on radiographs because the depth of the caries lies in a geometric plane that is not recorded radiographically (Fig. 14-4).

Fig. 14-4. Buccal caries as indicated by arrows. List the other carious lesions seen on these films.

Fig. 14-5. Interproximal caries.

Fig. 14-6. Diagram illustrating effect of contact point on caries interpretation.

Interproximal caries. The first sign of interproximal caries is a notching of the enamel, usually just below the contact point. As the caries progresses inward, it assumes a triangular shape, with the apex of the triangle toward the dentoenamel junction. As it invades the dentin, the caries spreads along the dentoenamel junction and proceeds toward the pulp in a roughly triangular-shaped pattern (Fig. 14-5).

The radiographic appearance of interproximal caries will be affected by the size and shape of the contact of the tooth involved. A tooth with a broad contact point will not show the caries as well as one with a narrow contact point because of the greater density of the tooth structure surrounding the caries (Fig. 14-6).

Conditions resembling caries

There are many radiolucencies seen on dental radiographs that may be mistaken for caries. The final diagnosis of caries is always made by corroborating the clinical examination with the radiographic findings.

Cervical burnout. Cervical burnout appears as a radiolucent band at the necks of the teeth. It is contrasted because the part of the tooth apical to it is covered by bone and hence more radiopaque and the area of the tooth occlusal to it is covered by enamel and is also radiopaque. In addition to these differences in densities caused by enamel and bone, the concave root contours below the cementoenamel junction will appear as radiolucencies. Cervical burnout is most often observed when there has been no loss of the alveolar bone that provides the radiographic contrast. It is seen most often in the mandibular incisors and molars (Fig. 14-7).

A

Fig. 14-7. Cervical burnout *(arrows)*. Anterior teeth also show pulp denticle, *a.*

B

Abrasions and attrition. Radiographically, cervical abrasion may resemble caries because it causes a wearing away of root structure and results in a decrease in density in the affected area. The radiolucency produced by the abrasion is usually a well-defined horizontal defect seen at the cementoenamel junction. Evidence of secondary dentin formation and pulp recession in response to the irritant may also be seen radiographically (Fig. 14-8). Attrition, which is defined as occlusal wear on teeth, can be seen clinically and radiographically.

Fig. 14-8. A, Attrition; **B,** Abrasion.

Fig. 14-9. Indirect pulp capping. Note radiolucent area under restoration in maxillary second molar.

Indirect pulp capping. A radiolucent shadow under a metallic restoration may not always indicate recurrent decay but an indirect pulp capping. To avoid a carious pulp exposure in this technique, the last remaining portion of decayed tooth is not excavated. A sedative base and permanent restoration are then placed with the hope that secondary dentin will be laid down to protect the pulp. Radiographically, the indirect pulp-capping procedure will show the radiolucent band of the unexcavated decay near the pulp chamber with a sedative base and permanent restoration (Fig. 14-9).

Restorative materials. Restorative materials such as silicates, acrylics, and some composites may resemble caries radiographically (Fig. 14-10). Recently some brands of composite filling material have had radiopaque materials added to their formulation (Fig. 14-11). Differentiation from caries of the radiolucent filling can be made on the basis of the regular geometric outline of a cavity preparation and the presence of a radiopaque cement base. All base and pulp-capping formulations that have a metallic component (e.g., zinc oxyphosphate, zinc oxide, calcium hydroxide) will appear radiopaque (Fig 14-12).

Fig. 14-10. Radiolucent restorations in central incisors.

Fig. 14-11. Radiopaque restorations mesial of central incisors.

Fig. 14-12. Radiopaque base and pulpotomy under metallic restoration.

PERIODONTAL DISEASE

The proper diagnosis and evaluation of periodontal disease can only be made with a combination of radiographic and clinical examinations. Periodontal disease has both soft tissue and bone components; there are radiographic limitations in both aspects of the disease process. Soft tissue (gingival) changes such as inflammation, hypertrophy, and recession will not be seen radiographically, since all soft tissue is radiolucent. Bone loss in some areas may not be seen because of superimpositions of buccal and lingual alveolar bone. It is helpful to remember that the radiograph portrays a three-dimensional disease process in two planes. Radiographic images of bone changes will almost always show less bone loss than there is.

Realizing these limitations, it is still important to remember that a proper periodontal diagnosis cannot be made without a full-mouth survey of radiographs. Radiographs serve to (1) identify predisposing factors, (2) detect early to moderate bone changes where treatment can preserve the dentition, (3) approximate the amount of bone loss and its location, (4) help in evaluating the prognosis of affected teeth and the restorative needs of these teeth, and (5) serve as baseline data and as a means of evaluating posttreatment results.

Techniques

The paralleling technique with a 16-inch focal-film distance is the best method for evaluating periodontal disease. A full periapical survey taken in this manner and augmented by either posterior, anterior, or vertical bite-wings is the technique of choice.

The use of the bisecting technique with its inherent dimensional distortion will give a distorted representation of the level of bone present (see Fig. 7-7).

Panoramic films are of little or no value in the diagnosis of periodontal disease except in the most advanced cases. Panoramic films should only be used if intraoral films cannot be taken.

Xeroradiography is an excellent imaging system to use in detecting periodontal disease. Soft tissue images are seen well and the wider range of densities will show early bone changes as well as small, less calcified calculus formation.

Predisposing factors

The detection of predisposing factors is one of the most important roles of radiography in periodontal disease. The treatment or prevention of early periodontal disease is much easier and has a higher success rate than efforts made once the disease has progressed further. The detection and elimination of local irritants are essential steps in prevention or actual periodontal therapy.

Calculus. Both subgingival and supragingival calculus are the most common of all local irritants. Early deposits, small and not fully calcified, will not be seen radiographically. Even when calcified, supragingival calculus, which is seen most often on the lingual surface of lower anterior teeth and the buccal surface of upper molars, will not be seen clearly in its early stage because of superimposition of tooth structure (Fig. 14-13). Subgingival calculus on the proximal surfaces is more easily detected in the early calcified stages. The calculus is seen as an irregularly pointed radiopaque projection from the proximal root surfaces (Fig. 14-14).

Fig. 14-13. Supragingival calculus on lingual surfaces of lower incisors.

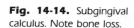

Fig. 14-14. Subgingival calculus. Note bone loss.

Restorations. Radiographic examination will reveal restorations with open contacts, poor contours, overhanging and deficient margins, and caries, all of which are etiologic factors in periodontal disease (Figs. 14-15 to 14-17).

Fig. 14-15. Over contoured crown on premolar and bone response.

Fig. 14-16. Restoration with open contact and overhang. Note bony response.

Fig. 14-17. Restoration with overhang. Note heavy calculus formation in other areas.

Fig. 14-18. Crown-root ratio—unfavorable.

Fig. 14-19. Early periodontal bone loss. Note fading of density of the alveolar crest, slight cupping, and triangulation.

Anatomic configurations. Only through radiographic examination can information about the size, shape, and position of the roots of periodontally involved teeth be obtained. These factors are important in evaluating the present condition and planning periodontal and restorative therapy.

The crown-root ratio refers to the length of root surface imbedded in bone compared with the length of the rest of the tooth. The greater the length of the tooth imbedded in bone, the better the prognosis (Fig. 14-18).

Teeth that have an anatomically short root will have a poorer prognosis periodontally than those teeth with long roots. Teeth with bulbous roots will have more area for attachment than those with fine, tapered roots. In multi-rooted teeth, the space between the roots is important; teeth with widely spaced roots have a better periodontal prognosis. Adjoining teeth whose roots are close together have a poorer prognosis than those with adequate areas of interseptal bone.

Gingivitis. Since gingivitis is a soft tissue change, there are no radiographic findings other than the presence of predisposing factors.

Radiographically detectable periodontal changes

Early (Fig. 14-19). This stage of periodontal change is characterized radiographically by changes in the crest of the interproximal bone septum and triangulation of the periodontal membrane. Triangulation is the widening of the periodontal membrane space at the crest of the interproximal septum that gives the appearance of a radiolucent triangle to what is normally a radiolucent band. The normal crest of the interseptal bone runs parallel to a line drawn between cementoenamel junctions on adjoining teeth at a level 1.0 to 1.5 mm below the cementoenamel junction. The crest of the septa will normally have a distinct radiopaque border. Fading of the density of the crest with cup-shaped defects is seen in the early stages of periodontal disease.

Moderate. In this stage bone loss is seen in both horizontal and vertical planes. Radiolucencies appear in the furcations of multirooted teeth, indicating bone loss in these critical areas (Fig. 14-20). Horizontal bone loss is resorption that occurs in a plane parallel to a line drawn between the cementoenamel junctions on adjoining teeth (Fig. 14-21). In vertical bone loss the resorption on

Fig. 14-20. Moderate to advanced bone loss showing bifurcation involvement.

Fig. 14-21. Horizontal bone loss.

Fig. 14-22. Vertical and horizontal bone loss. Note the early bifurcation involvement on the second molar.

Fig. 14-23. Different levels of buccal and lingual bone as indicated by arrows.

one tooth root sharing the septum is greater than on the other tooth, the so-called infra-bony pocket (Fig. 14-22). It is in this stage that horizontal bone loss on the buccal or lingual surfaces may go undetected because of superimposition. Careful examination of the radiograph may reveal a difference in density indicating different levels of bone on the buccal and lingual surfaces (Fig. 14-23).

Advanced (Figs. 14-24 and 14-25). This stage of periodontal disease is easily identified radiographically by the advanced vertical and horizontal bone loss, furcation involvement, thickened periodontal membranes, and indications of changes in tooth position.

Fig. 14-24. Advanced periodontal bone loss.

Fig. 14-25. Trifurcation bone loss upper first molar; bifurcation bone loss lower first and second molar.

Periodontal abscess (Fig. 14-26). The radiographic signs of a periodontal abscess vary greatly. To make such a diagnosis, there must be an acute clinical manifestation. Periodontal abscess is caused by the occlusion of an existing pocket; therefore the radiograph of the acute episode may not vary greatly from previous films of the existing condition that produced the pocket. In other instances there may be signs of rapid and extensive bone destruction.

Fig. 14-26. Periodontal abscess. Patient had acute buccal swelling and facial edema.

Fig. 14-27. Pulp chambers receded with age. Secondary dentin formation.

PULPAL LESIONS

High pulp horns and large pulp chambers can occur in all age groups, not just in the young patients of which these findings are characteristic. The normal size and shape of the pulp chamber and canals change with age, in certain developmental anomalies as dentinogenesis imperfecta, and in response to local irritants. Gradual reduction is marked by the deposition of secondary dentin at the walls of the chamber and canals (Fig. 14-27). Radiographically, secondary

Fig. 14-28. Secondary dentin formation in second molar in response to caries and restoration.

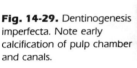

Fig. 14-29. Dentinogenesis imperfecta. Note early calcification of pulp chamber and canals.

and regular dentin appear the same and can only be differentiated by the changes in the shape of the chamber and canals that accompany aging. The formation of secondary dentin with the resulting obliteration or narrowing of the pulp chamber and canals can be caused by different types of irritants. The most common causes are deep caries, pulp capping, deep-seated restorations, attrition, abrasion, and a healed tooth fracture (Fig. 14-28). This decrease in pulp and root chamber size is also seen in the developmental disturbances dentinogenesis imperfecta and dentinal dysplasia (Fig. 14-29).

Pulp stones or calcifications appear as well-defined radiopacities within the pulp chamber (Fig. 14-30). A radiolucent line may be seen separating the stone from the pulpal wall or it may be attached to the floor or wall of the chamber. The stones, which are composed of either dentin or calcified salts, will have the density and appearance of dentin.

Fig. 14-30. Pulp stones in lower incisors.

Fig. 14-31. Pulpitis with no apical changes. Second premolar was acutely sensitive to thermal stimulation and was found to be partially nonvital.

Pulpitis

There are no radiographic signs of pulpitis in the pulp chamber. Normal, inflamed, or necrotic pulp all appear the same, because their densities are the same. The only possible radiographic findings in pulpitis are the causative factors such as caries, pulp exposure, previous pulp capping, or deep restorations (Fig. 14-31). The pulps of teeth may vary in radiographic density. This is not because of differences in vitality but because of the differences in object density of the overlying tooth structure.

PERIAPICAL LESIONS

Periapical lesions are seen in the apical tissues surrounding the tooth after the pulp has become necrotic. The periodontal membrane, lamina dura, and alveolar bone are the affected tissues. This necrosis, or degeneration of the pulp, may be a result of carious invasion of the pulp or physical or chemical trauma. The exudate from the pulp first spills into the periodontal ligament, causing a thickening that can be seen radiographically (Fig. 14-32). The pressure then causes resorption of the lamina dura and alveolar bone. Depending on certain factors, a cyst, granuloma, or dentoalveolar abscess may develop at this point. It is almost impossible to differentiate radiographically between a periapical cyst and a periapical granuloma (Figs. 14-33 and 14-34). The dentoalveolar abscess may cause root resorption and a more diffuse radiolucency (Fig. 14-35). A fistulous track leading from the abscess to the oral cavity, if present, is very difficult to see on radiographs because of its tortuous course.

Fig. 14-32. Thickened periodontal membrane and early apical bone change on maxillary cuspid.

Fig. 14-33. Periapical granuloma.

Fig. 14-34. Periapical cyst.

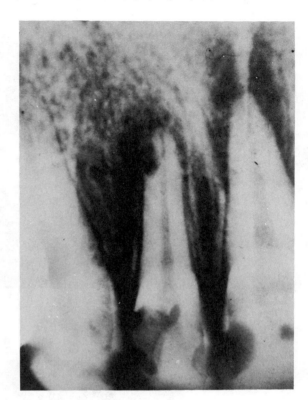

Fig. 14-35. Dentoalveolar abscess.

Periapical condensing osteitis

Periapical condensing osteitis is recognized by the formation of dense bone around the apex of a tooth in response to low-grade pulpal necrosis. This asymptomatic condition is seen most often at the mandibular premolar and molar apices (Fig. 14-36). In almost all cases the teeth are shown to be nonvital through testing. Although the tooth may be asymptomatic, it should be looked on as a radiopaque type of periapical pathologic condition and treated accordingly.

Residual periapical lesions

Residual periapical lesions are radiolucencies in either the maxilla or the mandible. They represent areas of pathology that arose from teeth that were extracted in the area. If a granuloma or cyst that surrounds the apex of a nonvital tooth is not curetted out at the time of extraction, it may remain and grow and is considered either a residual cyst or a granuloma (Fig. 14-37).

Fig. 14-36. Periapical condensing osteitis on mesial and distal roots of first molar.

Fig. 14-37. Residual cyst of mandible.

Fig. 14-38. Hypercementosis. Note club shaped root on second premolar.

Hypercementosis

Hypercementosis is a condition characterized by the buildup of cementum on the root of the tooth. Normally it is difficult to distinguish cementum from dentin because of its thin layers. The buildup of cementum makes the root appear "club" shaped instead of its usual conical appearance (Fig. 14-38). This condition is often associated with non-vital teeth and is seen in patients who have Paget's disease of bone.

Root resorption

Root resorption can be caused by chronic periapical or periodontal infection, trauma, pressure from tumors or cysts, or rapid excessive orthodontic pressure, or it can be idiopathic (Figs. 14-39 to 14-42).

Internal resorption (Fig. 14-43). The cause of this internally destructive process is unknown. The radiographic findings of internal resorption are irregularities and widening of the usually smooth, tapered outline of the root chamber. In advanced cases the irregular outline of the resorption can be seen perforating the root and reaching the periodontal ligament.

External resorption (Fig. 14-44). The cause of this resorptive process is also unknown. Radiographically, teeth with external resorption will have a round or oval radiolucency lateral to or superimposed over the pulp canal. If it is superimposed, the outline of the normal canal can be seen through the superimposition. If the radiolucency is lateral to the pulp canal, it will not in its early stages communicate with the pulp canal but in it's later stages will perforate.

Fig. 14-39. Root resorption resulting from trauma.

Fig. 14-40. Root resorption resulting from chronic periodontal infection.

Fig. 14-41. Root resorption resulting from excessive and rapid orthodontic movement.

Fig. 14-42. Root resorption resulting from a malignant tumor.

Fig. 14-43. Internal root resorption.

Fig. 14-44. External root resorption.

Fig. 14-45. Cementoma; all teeth test vital.

Cementoma (fibro-osteoma) (PCD—periapical cemental dysplasia) (Fig. 14-45)

Cementoma is a three-stage lesion that is asymptomatic and self-limiting and for which there is no treatment indicated. It occurs at the apical region, and it originates in the periodontal membrane of the tooth. In its first stage it is radiolucent and resembles periapical disease. The second stage is mixed, because the radiolucent lesion starts to calcify. In its third stage it is totally radiopaque. Clinically the teeth always test vital.

TRAUMATIC INJURIES

Fractures of teeth, especially anterior teeth, are very common. Clinically and radiographically, a fracture of the crown of a tooth is easier to detect than a root fracture. The fracture will be seen on the radiograph as a radiolucent line, or the missing part of the tooth will be apparent (Fig. 14-46). A root fracture is also seen as a radiolucent line but is much more difficult to visualize because of superimposition of alveolar bone trabeculation (Fig. 14-47). Fractures of the maxilla and mandible maybe seen in part on periapical film, but larger views such as panoramic or extraoral are needed for complete visualization (Figs. 14-48 and 14-49).

Fig. 14-46. Fractured crowns of maxillary central incisors. Note proximity of fracture lines to pulp chambers.

Fig. 14-47. Root fracture of maxillary central incisor.

Fig. 14-48. Panoramic radiograph showing fractured mandible.

Fig. 14-49. Fracture of mandible on a lateral oblique film.

FOREIGN BODIES AND ROOT TIPS

It is possible to have any sort of foreign body imbedded in the jawbones. Only those that are radiopaque will be seen radiographically. Metallic foreign bodies are the easiest to see and the most common. These radiopacities may be amalgam, burrs, broken instruments, needles, metallic fragments from an external source (Fig. 14-50), or metallic implants (Fig. 14-51).

Retained root tips will have the density of tooth structure (Fig. 14-52). It is sometimes very difficult to distinguish between the retained root tip and dense areas of bone. One way to differentiate between the root tip and dense bone areas is the appearance of a pulp canal or the conical shape of a root tip. These root tips should be localized radiographically in three dimensions before surgery is attempted.

Fig. 14-50. Metallic foreign body in mandible.

Fig. 14-51. Metallic implant of the mandible serving as distal abutment. Note thinning of bone indicating start of rejection process.

Fig. 14-52. Retained root tip in maxillary molar region.

Fig. 14-53. Extraction socket in mandible.

EXTRACTION SOCKETS

Extraction sockets may be radiographically evident in the bone up to 6 months after surgery. The area eventually fills in with bone in the normal trabecular pattern (Fig. 14-53).

CYSTS AND TUMORS

All cysts located in bone will be seen as radiolucent areas. Tumors can appear either radiolucent or radiopaque. When the cyst and the tumor appear radiolucent, it is because the lesion has destroyed normal bone and replaced it with less-dense cystic or tumor tissue (Fig. 14-54). If the lesion is radiopaque, this signifies that the new tumor tissue being formed has a greater density or size than the tissue it is replacing (Fig. 14-55). Tumors of bone and cartilage will appear radiopaque, while all other tumors will appear radiolucent. It is mandatory for the diagnostician to be able to see the entire lesion and be able to define its borders and extent in three planes before any type of treatment is instituted.

The possibility of malignancy must always be kept in mind when diagnosing an unknown lesion. In general, malignancies tend to have poorly defined radiographic borders and will destroy normal anatomic structures (Fig. 14-56). Benign tumors and cysts will expand slowly with clearly defined borders. Their

Fig. 14-54. Radiograph of tumor (ameloblastoma) enveloping teeth.

Fig. 14-55. Panoramic radiograph showing well-defined radiopaque tumor in left maxillary sinus. Compare right and left maxillary sinuses.

Fig. 14-56. Lateral oblique radiograph showing destruction of coronoid process by malignant tumor.

A

B

Fig. 14-57. A, Occlusal radiograph showing expansion of buccal and lingual plates of mandible caused by benign tumor. B, Occlusal radiograph showing perforation and spread through the buccal and lingual cortices by a malignant tumor.

slow growth tends to displace rather than destroy structures. On occlusal films benign lesions will expand the buccal and lingual cortex of bone, while malignant lesions will perforate and invade neighboring tissue (Fig. 14-57).

In large pathologic areas it will be necessary to use the accessory techniques described in Chapter 9 to visualize the entire lesion and to make a radiographic diagnosis.

METABOLIC BONE LESIONS

Many metabolic diseases will manifest themselves with changes of the trabecular pattern and lamina dura of bone in the mandible and maxilla. Examples of this type of disease process would be Paget's disease, hyperparathyroidism, and certain types of anemia. It is not the role of the dental auxiliary to be able to diagnose these diseases, but rather to be able to recognize the changes seen on the radiographs (Figs. 14-58 to 14-60).

Fig. 14-58. Paget's disease. Lateral skull projection showing the characteristic "cotton wool" appearance of Paget's disease of bone.

Fig. 14-59. Radiolucent lesion of hyperparathyroidism seen between roots of premolars.

Fig. 14-60. Trabecular bone pattern of anemia. Note enlarged medullary spaces.

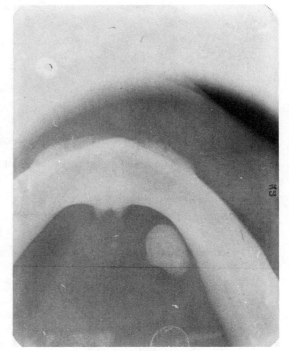

Fig. 14-61. Occlusal radiograph of edentulous mandible showing radiopaque salivary stone in submandibular duct in floor of mouth.

Fig. 14-62. Salivary stone seen on panoramic film (stone is seen twice because of redundant image).

SALIVARY STONES

Although not a bone lesion, salivary stones are included here because salivary gland disease is often treated by the dentist. Although the salivary glands and ducts are soft tissue, radiographs are still important in the diagnostic workup. Salivary stones (sialoliths) are a common cause of obstruction, secondary swelling, and infection. Since the sialolith is calcified, it can be detected on radiographs. Stones in the submandibular duct can best be seen on a mandibular occlusal film (Fig. 14-61). Stones can also be seen on panoramic and lateral oblique film (Fig. 14-62). For the parotid gland, in which stones are not so common, a lateral oblique, posteroanterior, or soft tissue film placed in the muccobuccal fold can be employed.

15

Legal considerations

It may be a sign of our times, but no discussion of a subject in the health sciences can be considered complete today without mentioning the legal aspects that affect the profession. Radiology is no exception and is probably the most regulated discipline within dentistry. We must therefore understand the laws and regulations, both local and federal, that govern the use of radiation in our profession.

The legal considerations with which the dental auxiliary should be familiar regarding the use of ionizing radiation in dentistry fall into three major categories: (1) federal and state regulations regarding x-ray equipment and its use, (2) licensure for users of x-ray equipment, and (3) risk management.

FEDERAL AND STATE REGULATIONS

All dental x-ray machines either manufactured or sold in the United States after 1974 must meet the federal government's performance standards, which include safety specifications for minimum filtration and accuracy and reproduceability of the milliamperage time and kilovoltage settings. These standards were discussed in Chapters 1 and 2.

All x-ray equipment, regardless of date of manufacture, is also subject to state, county, or city radiation health codes. These codes can also include regulations concerning barriers, film speed, and position of the operator. It is not unusual for registration of x-ray machines to be required and a fee charged for such a permit.

Many states or other jurisdictions require biannual or triennial inspections of the x-ray machines and the dental office, for which a fee is charged. Violations of the radiation code can lead to fines or suspension of a dentist's radiation permit. The positive aspect of these inspections is that they serve as a quality assurance (QA) procedure. The inspectors as they measure for violations are performing recommended QA procedures.

LICENSURE

Each state will have its own policy for the user of dental radiation. The dental hygienist, who in all states is a licensed person, may or may not have to take an additional examination to be certified to take radiographs. The dental assistant may be required to take a radiology examination other than the national certifying examination to be able to take dental radiographs. Some states have exceptions in their radiation rules that allow an uncertified dental assistant to take radiographs under the direct supervision of a dentist. Direct supervision means that the dentist is physically present in the office when the radiographs are being taken. In some states dental assistants cannot take extraoral films other than a panoramic film.

Each state deals with dental radiography differently. It is not the purpose of this text to compile lists of these requirements, because they are constantly changing. The dental auxiliary should be knowledgeable about the rules and regulations of the state or jurisdiction in which one is working and should not assume that all state regulations are the same.

RISK MANAGEMENT

By far the most important legal aspect of dental radiology is risk management. We all know about the increase in the number of malpractice suits against health professionals. Dentistry has not been excluded from this trend, and malpractice actions have increased in number and amount of awards over the recent years. Risk management is the policies and procedures that will reduce the likelihood of suits for malpractice against dentists. All members of the dental staff must be aware and participate in these programs if they are to be effective.

First, let it be made clear that the liability, both professionally and legal, rests with the dentist and not the dental hygienist or the dental assistant. This is called the *doctrine of respondeat superior* or "captain of the ship" principle; more simply put, the captain of the ship is responsible for the actions of the sailors. The auxiliary may be named in a lawsuit, but the liability is with the employing dentist.

A dental hygienist falls under the doctrine of respondeat superior if she or he is an employee. If the hygienist is the one found to be negligent, the dentist's insurance company may decide to subrogate the payment of the claim against the hygienist or the hygienist's insurance company. Therefore it is advisable for the hygienist to carry professional liability insurance. If the hygienist is an independent contractor, then he or she may be sued alone. What then is the role of the dental auxiliary in a risk management program?

Patient relations

Avoiding misunderstandings is very important and an essential to risk management. The patient should be told in advance what the office policy is in regard to financial arrangements, payments, recall procedures and the filing of insurance claims.

One should never say anything negative about anything relating to equipment procedures or staff. If the equipment is not working correctly, one should not complain in front of or to the patient. Remarks such as "This timer is always off" or "These films weren't processed properly" are unnecessary. These are considered to be "admissions against interest" or the theory of *res gestae*. Statements made by anyone spontaneously at the time of an alleged negligent act are admissible as evidence.

Informed consent

The dental auxiliary should participate in the process of obtaining informed consent. This is explaining to the patient the nature and purpose of the procedure, in this case the taking of radiographs, in lay terms and clarifying the risks and benefits to be derived. It is equally important, and recent legal decisions have said, that the patient must be informed of the risks of not having a specific procedure. In this case the patient must be told about the diseases that might go undetected without radiographs and what the consequences might be. If the patient is a minor, the parent or guardian must give the consent.

Health questionnaire

The dental auxillary should always review the health questionnaire and update it where necessary. One should call to the dentist's attention any information that might contraindicate or change the number and type of radiographs that are to be taken.

RECORDS

It has been said that the three most important parts of a defense in a malpractice suit are "records, records, records." Dental radiographs are considered part of the patient's dental record and so are considered to be legal documents. The quality of the radiographs may be an important issue in any litigation. If the quality is poor and nondiagnostic and the procedures in question are based on the radiographs, this substantially weakens the defense. If the radiographs are lost or misfiled or do not have archival life, then again the case for the defense is seriously compromised. One can readily recognize the role of the dental auxiliary in this phase of risk management.

The patient's records are confidential. The contents or the findings in these records should never be discussed or shown to anyone outside of the office. This includes any radiographs or photographs that are part of the record.

OWNERSHIP

Radiographs are the property of the dentist. Patients may request a copy of their radiographs. This request should be written and signed by the patient. A fee may be charged for this duplication. Laws differ from state to state on whether you must give the radiographs to the patient if the fee for this service has not been paid. In some states the radiographs must be given to the patient even if the fee has not been paid. The dentist may pursue collection, but only after giving the radiographs to the patient. This is not true in all states and only goes to emphasize the point that one must be familiar with the laws regulating practice in the state in which one works.

The dentist should be informed of this request and an entry made in the record of when and to whom the radiographs were sent. Never under any circumstances should the original radiographs be given or sent to a patient. There is no defense if there are no radiographs. One should not make the assumption that "This is an old and loyal patient who would never dream of legal action." That is a poor risk management assumption.

Retention. Dental radiographs should be kept for 7 years after the patient ceases to be a patient. Ideally they should be kept forever. Actions that can be brought against a dentist depend on the statue of limitations. The usual time limitation for an adult is 3 years after the discovery of the injury or when the injury should have been discovered. For children it is 3 years after they reach their majority, which in some states is 21. Suits therefore can be brought many years past the mandated 7 years of retention of radiographs.

INSURANCE CLAIMS

It is the legitimate right of the insurance company to request copies of pretreatment radiographs to evaluate the treatment plan. The original radiographs should never be sent to the insurance company, because they may be lost in the mail or by the insurance company. In either case the dentist is left without an important part of the patient's record, and in case of litigation the fact that the originals were lost is no defense.

As mentioned previously, radiographs should never be taken to prove to the insurance company that the services have been performed. This would be an administrative radiograph.

Appendix

Study questions

1. What are radiations? Explain the differences between two types of radiations used in diagnostic imaging.
2. Explain the differences and similarities between radio waves and x-rays.
3. Identify the parts of the dental x-ray tube labeled *A* through *I* in Fig. A-1 and give the function of each part.
4. List the controls present on the control panel of a dental x-ray machine and what each determines.
5. Explain the difference between filtration and collimation of the x-ray beam. What are the requirements of each?
6. What is rectangular collimation? Why is it important?
7. Explain the difference between kilovoltage and milliamperage and what they control in the dental x-ray machine.
8. What is ionization? Describe how x-rays produce ionization.
9. What are the types of transformers used in a dental x-ray machine, and what is their function?
10. Do walls and equipment in dental operatories become radioactive after many years of absorbing x-rays? Explain.
11. Do all the x-ray photons produced at the cathode have the same energy? Why? If not, what is done to correct this condition?
12. Identify the parts of the dental x-ray machine seen in Fig. A-2.
13. What is the thermionic emission effect? At what point in the x-ray tube does it occur?
14. What determines the penetrating power of the x-rays? How is this controlled?
15. What does the milliamperage determine?
16. Explain the concept of milliampere seconds.
17. Why is there a need for filtration of the x-ray beam?
18. Why are exposure times now expressed in impulses rather than fractions of seconds?
19. What is the disadvantage of using a closed-end, pointed cone?
20. How would you describe the size of the x-ray beam relative to the size of the intraoral film?
21. Explain the following terms and sketch examples of each: (a) object-film distance, (b) focal-film distance, and (c) divergent and parallel rays of the x-ray beam.
22. What factors determine the density and contrast of the finished radiograph?
23. What is the ideal relationship for intraoral radiography between the x-ray tube, tooth, and film packet? Can this be achieved? Why or why not?
24. What is the importance of target (focal) area size?
25. Does the patient receive greater exposure to radiation with the longer exposures in the 16-inch FFD when compared with a comparable radiograph using an 8-inch FFD?
26. What determines film speed? What film speed should be used?
27. What is the purpose of the lead foil in the film packet?

Fig. A-1

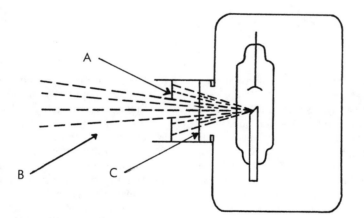

Fig. A-2

28. What is film fog? What are its causes?
29. Explain the inverse square law. Give two clinical applications of its use.
30. What are the three types of movement that can cause loss of detail?
31. Why is a focal film distance of greater than 16 inches not recommended?
32. Explain the difference between a double emulsion film and a double film packet.
33. What would be the result of using a focal-film distance of less than 8 inches?
34. What is the recessed tube? What is its purpose?
35. Explain the difference between long-scale and short-scale contrast. By what are they determined?
36. Explain what the ANSI classification of dental film means.
37. What are the advantages of the 16-inch focal film distance technique when compared with the 8-inch technique?

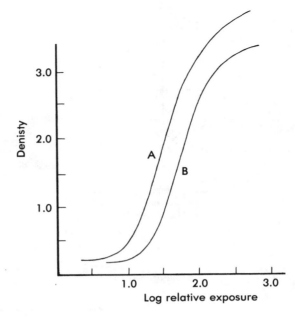

Fig. A-3

38. Name three imaging systems used in dentistry today.
39. When changing from an 8-inch focal film distance to a 16-inch one, what changes, if any, must be made to the lead diaphragm?
40. What are the indications for using a double film pack?
41. In Fig. A-3 which film, *A* or *B,* requires less exposure time for intraoral exposures?
42. What is the primary mechanism for tissue change resulting from dental x-ray exposure?
43. Explain the difference between the terms *exposure* and *dose*.
44. What is the difference between a roentgen, a rad, and a rem?
45. What is a dose response curve? What type is applicable in radiation dosage?
46. What is the output of an x-ray machine? How is it measured?
47. What are the units for measuring radiation based on the metric system? How do these units relate to the conventional system?

48. How much background radiation does the population of the United States receive each year? What are the major sources of this background radiation?
49. Explain the difference between a localized dose and total body dose.
50. What body cells are most sensitive to ionizing radiation?
51. Approximately what is the facial exposure from a full-mouth x-ray survey? How is it calculated?
52. Explain the risk-versus-benefit concept.
53. What does the latent period refer to in radiation?
54. What may be some of the long-term effects of radiation?
55. How does one make risk estimates for radiation?
56. Name some risks encountered in everyday living that compare with the risks of developing cancer from dental radiation.
57. What is the erythema dose for skin? Is it important or a danger in dental radiography?

58. How does one handle the dental radiographic needs of a pregnant patient?
59. Is the dose rate an important factor in tissue reaction to radiation? Why?
60. What is the rule of ALARA?
61. Explain the differences between primary and secondary radiation.
62. How do federal and state regulations differ in regard to dental radiology?
63. Explain the effect of kVp on patient dosage.
64. What is the disadvantage with mechanical timers?
65. What is the best type of position-indicating device?
66. What is the advantage of using group E film? Is there a disadvantage? Explain.
67. Why is the paralleling technique preferred over the bisecting technique in regard patient dosage?
68. What is the relationship between focal-film distance and patient dosage?
69. What does the term *selection criteria* mean? Give some examples.
70. Explain what is meant by the maximum permissible dose for dental personnel. What is its present value?
71. What are administrative radiographs? What is their present status?
72. Where should the operator be positioned when taking radiographs?
73. Is it permissible for dental personnel to hold films in a handicapped patient's mouth while x-ray exposures are made?
74. What constitutes adequate shielding in the dental office? Are lead walls mandatory?
75. What are the advantages of wearing film badges?
76. How is patient shielding accomplished?
77. Can pregnant dental personnel continue to take radiographs during pregnancy?
78. What is the importance of the patient's radiation history?
79. Name the components of an office quality assurance program that would fall into the realm of responsibility of the dental auxiliary.
80. List six major ways to reduce x-ray dose for patients.
81. List the ways that the operator dose can be kept to zero.
82. In dental radiology what are the main vectors for cross-contamination?
83. What are the required barriers that dental personnel must wear during all radiographic procedures?
84. What are some of the barriers that can be used for equipment and the operatory in dental radiology?
85. What is the difference between sterilization and disinfection? Where is each used in dental radiology?
86. What diseases should dental personnel receive immunization for?
87. Do the processing solutions used in the darkroom act as sterilizing agents for the film?
88. What is the cross-contamination hazard with daylight loaders?
89. List the infection control procedures that should be followed before, during, and after taking dental radiographs.
90. List and describe the steps in the processing of dental x-ray film and the purpose of each.
91. What is a safelight? How do you test for reliability?
92. What is the time-temperature technique?
93. What is sight developing? Is it an acceptable technique?
94. Why is underdeveloping to compensate for overexposure not an acceptable technique?
95. List the chemicals that make up the developer and fixer solutions and the function of each.
96. What are the clinical indications for rapid processing? What are its disadvantages?
97. When must safelight conditions be maintained in the darkroom?
98. What are the dental auxiliary's responsibilities in the darkroom?
99. Distinguish between cone cutting and developer cutoff.

100. Can one distinguish between an overexposed film and an overdeveloped film? How?
101. What can cause a clear film?
102. Discuss the importance of a quality assurance program in the darkroom.
103. When should processing solutions be changed?

104. What will happen if film is left in the fixer solution over a weekend?
105. How are x-ray films duplicated?
106. Give two indications for the need for duplicate films.
107. A duplicate film series comes out too dark. List two ways to correct this error.

Metallic filling
Pulp
Caries
Dentin
Enamel
Air

Fig. A-4

108. Describe the methods for testing the strength of the processing solutions.
109. What are unibath solutions?
110. What stages of the developing process are seen diagrammatically in Fig. A-4, 2 and 3?
111. Explain the difference between a periapical and bite-wing film. What is the use of each?
112. List the criteria that determine whether a radiograph is diagnostic.
113. Why is there less thyroid exposure in the paralleling technique than in the bisecting technique?
114. What is a major concern in using nondisposable film holders?
115. Why is gagging no longer a factor in using longer focal-film distance?
116. Explain dimensional distortion and how it applies to the paralleling technique.
117. What is the advantage of an increased FFD (8 to 16 inches)?
118. What is parallel in the paralleling technique?
119. What is a localizing ring? What is its function?
120. Name some devices that can be used to hold film in the paralleling technique.
121. Can the paralleling technique be used with rectangular collimation?
122. Why is the paralleling technique superior to the bisecting technique in interpreting periodontal bone height?
123. Why is there no superimposition of the zygomatic arch on the apices of maxillary molars in the paralleling technique?
124. Can the paralleling technique be used with an 8-inch FFD?
125. What technique is always used in the bite-wing projection?
126. What is the proper chair position for radiography using the bisecting-angle technique? Is this necessary in the bisecting technique?
127. Explain the theory of the bisecting-angle technique.
128. What are the advantages and disadvantages of this technique?
129. What do the terms *point of entry*,

vertical angulation, and *horizontal angulation* mean?
130. Why is a full-mouth series of radiographs necessary for an edentulous patient?
131. What causes elongated and foreshortened images on radiographs?
132. What causes overlapping of images on radiographs?
133. What is the correct sagittal plane orientation for the patient's head? What errors are caused by poor orientation?
134. What determines the variations in degree of vertical angulation from projection to projection in the bisecting-angle technique?
135. What are two possible alternatives to a 13-film edentulous survey?
136. Explain why it is necessary to use occlusal films in localizing impacted teeth. Are there any other ways to localize impactions?
137. List three indications for using extraoral views in dentistry.
138. Which extraoral projection is most diagnostic for pathologic conditions of the maxillary sinus? How is this film taken?
139. What extra precautions must be taken in the darkroom when loading cassettes and processing extraoral films?
140. What are the advantages of using rare earth intensifying screens?
141. How do rare earth intensifying screens differ from conventional calcium tungstate screens?
142. What will happen if an intensifying screen is accidentally scratched in the darkroom?
143. What purposes does a grid serve in extraoral projections?
144. How can one differentiate the left side of the patient from the right on an extraoral radiograph?
145. What projection would you use to localize a foreign body in the floor of the mouth?
146. What are the best ways to radiograph the temporomandibular joint with dental equipment?
147. How does the use of intensifying

screens reduce the exposure time needed for radiographs?

148. Why is correct positioning of the patient's head so important in pantomographic radiology?

149. If a periapical film of an impacted mandibular third molar cannot be positioned so the complete root can be seen, what would you do?

150. What areas of the maxilla and mandible are not shown clearly on the pantomographic radiograph?

151. Is a pantomographic or a bite-wing film more diagnostic for caries? Why?

152. Compare the patient dosage received in a full-mouth survey with that of a pantomogram.

153. What is the plane of acceptable detail? What is another name for it?

154. What are the advantages of panoramic films over intraoral periapicals?

155. What is the main disadvantage of panoramic films?

156. Name three anatomic structures seen on panoramic films that are not seen on an intraoral full mouth series.

157. How are panoramic films processed? Can they be processed in all automatic processors?

158. What technique error causes the spinal column to be superimposed on the ramus of the mandible?

159. Where should the patient's tongue be when one is making a panoramic exposure?

160. What causes static marks on the finished panoramic film?

161. What is the role of the dental auxiliary in patient management?

162. Describe the personal hygienic procedures in dental radiography of which the dental auxiliary should be aware.

163. How can the dental auxiliary convey a feeling of confidence to the patient?

164. What do you do in a situation in which a patient refuses to be radiographed?

165. Why is it important for the dental auxiliary to be able to discuss radiation hazards with the patient?

166. Outline some methods that may be employed to prevent patient gagging.

167. What is the usual problem in intraoral radiography of impacted maxillary and mandibular third molars?

168. Describe the three methods that can be used to localize an impaction.

169. Why is the shallow palate more of a problem in the paralleling technique than in the bisecting-angle technique?

170. What is the reverse bite-wing technique?

171. List some methods that might be used to orient a new child patient to the use of dental x-rays.

172. What is the proper film order when taking a full-mouth radiographic survey? Why?

173. What are some of the reasons that may make it impossible to take intraoral films?

174. If intraoral films cannot be taken, what should be done? Why?

175. Define *radiolucent* and *radiopaque*. Give an example of each.

176. What determines whether any object will be radiolucent or radiopaque?

177. In the labial mounting technique, what is the film orientation in relation to the viewer?

178. Radiographically, how could you differentiate the mandibular molar edentulous film from the maxillary molar edentulous film?

179. On what radiographic projection is the coronoid process of the mandible seen?

180. Why is the mental foramen seen as a radiolucency?

181. Which is the most radiopaque of the natural tooth structures? Which is the most radiolucent?

182. On what projections is the maxillary sinus seen?

183. Name two radiolucencies seen on the maxillary incisor radiograph.

184. Does the maxilla or the mandible have the denser trabecular pattern?

Fig. A-5

185. In which area are nutrient canals easiest to identify?
186. Radiographically, how could you differentiate a mandibular premolar film from a maxillary premolar film?
187. How and why do the lips, cheek, and nose affect the radiograph?
188. On which extraoral projections can the maxillary sinus be seen? Which is the best view for visualizing it?
189. Identify the dental, structures labeled *A* through *F* in Fig. A-5.
190. What is the role of the dental auxiliary in diagnosis?
191. Give an example of how error in technique can lead to a deficient diagnosis.
192. What is a supernumerary tooth, and what are its clinical consequences?
193. What is the clinical significance of hypodontia in the secondary dentition?
194. Distinguish between amelogenesis imperfecta and dentinogenesis imperfecta.

195. How can a radiographic examination help in evaluating tooth development and eruption?
196. Describe what teeth would be seen on a mandibular molar periapical film of a 10-year-old patient.
197. How does an impacted tooth appear radiographically?
198. Distinguish between concrescence and fusion.
199. Describe a dilacerated tooth.
200. How does a cleft palate appear radiographically?
201. What is the best radiographic projection to visualize a median palatal cyst?
202. Distinguish between a nasopalatine cyst and a globulomaxillary cyst in regard to radiographic appearance and location.
203. Describe the radiographic appearance of a dentigerous cyst.
204. Why is it important to localize impacted teeth in three planes?

Fig. A-6

205. Why do caries appear radiolucent on radiographs?
206. Name some other conditions found on radiographs that might be misinterpreted as caries.
207. Why is it difficult to visualize occlusal and buccal caries radiographically?
208. Identify the caries on the radiographs seen in Fig. A-6.
209. Name some predisposing factors to periodontal disease that can be seen on radiographs.
210. Describe the appearance of calculus on a radiograph. Is it always seen radiographically?
211. What are the radiographic signs of early periodontal disease? Of advanced periodontal disease?
212. Differentiate between internal and external idiopathic resorption.
213. Would the bite-wing film be the projection of choice for diagnosis of traumatic injury to teeth? Why?

214. Differentiate between hypercementosis and a cementoma.
215. What characterizes a malignant tumor radiographically?
216. Name some possible causes of root resorption.
217. What are the radiographic characteristics of a benign tumor?
218. Describe the radiographic appearance of condensing osteitis. How does it differ from a cementoma?
219. Why are cysts seen as radiolucencies?
220. In making the diagnosis of a necrotic pulp, why is it essential to be able to see the apex of the tooth on the radiograph?
221. What are sialoliths? How are they best radiographed?
222. Name three causes of root resorption.
223. How does a fracture appear radiographically? Why?

The following are released questions from the National Board Dental Hygiene Examination. Test yourself. The answers will be found at the end of the exercise.

1. Using an E speed rather than a D speed film to produce a radiograph requires:
   1. a longer exposure time
   2. a shorter exposure time
   3. the same exposure time
   4. a longer processing time
   5. a shorter processing time

2. The periodontal ligament surrounding a normal tooth appears radiographically as:
   1. an unbroken radiopaque line around the tooth root
   2. a radiopaque line on the lateral sides of the root only
   3. an unbroken radiolucent line around the tooth root
   4. a radiolucent line around the apical portion of the root only

3. Which of the following positions indicating devices best minimizes the dose of radiation to the patient?
   1. pointed, plastic
   2. leaded, circular
   3. open-ended circular
   4. leaded, rectangular

4. Which of the following materials is most effective in stopping x-rays?
   1. lead
   2. copper
   3. enamel
   4. tungsten
   5. aluminum

5. Each successive panoramic film appears lighter than the one before. Which of the following corrections should be made?
   1. increase the mA setting
   2. increase the kVp setting
   3. change the intensifying screens
   4. replenish the developer solution
   5. increase the temperature of the developer solution
   6. decrease the temperature of the developer solution

6. The rays that are most apt to be absorbed by the skin are the x-rays that are:

1. of short wave length
2. of long wave length
3. aluminum filtered
4. deep and penetrating

7. The speed at which electrons move across the tube is regulated by:
   1. kilovoltage
   2. milliamperage
   3. both (1) and (2)
   4. neither (1) nor (2)

8. Changing from 75 kVp to 90 kVp will:
   1. decrease radiographic density
   2. decrease radiographic contrast
   3. increase radiographic contrast
   4. increase radiographic exposure time

9. All teeth test vital in an 11-year-old patient. A radiolucency at the apices of a permanent mandibular second molar that has no caries or restorations is probably:
   1. a granuloma
   2. a residual cyst
   3. root resorption
   4. a periapical abscess
   5. incomplete root formation

10. For radiation, "MPD" stands for:
    1. minimize patient dose
    2. maximum permissible dose
    3. mutation potential dose
    4. manufacturer's patented dose
    5. maintain perfect documentation

11. In a periapical radiograph, the major change caused by increasing the vertical angle when using the bisecting-angle technique is:
    1. elongation
    2. overlapping
    3. foreshortening
    4. apical shifting of the image

12. Which of the following allows for greater penetration of x-rays?
    1. increased kVp
    2. decreased kVp
    3. increased amperage
    4. decreased amperage
    5. increased exposure time

13. In developing radiographs, the fixer acts to:

1. prevent film fog and soften the emulsion
2. remove exposed silver halide and soften the emulsion
3. remove exposed silver halide and shrink and harden the emulsion
4. remove unexposed and undeveloped silver halide from the emulsion and rehardens the emulsion

14. Which of the following structures appear radiolucent on a radiograph?
   1. nares, median suture, medullary spaces
   2. incisive canal, genial tubercles, nasal fossa
   3. maxillary sinus, mylohyoid ridge, mental foramen
   4. hamular process, nutrient canals, nasal cartilage
   5. coronoid process, mandibular canal, maxillary septum

15. Which of the following anatomic structures is usually *not* demonstrated on intraoral periapical radiographs?
   1. mental foramen
   2. mylohyoid ridge
   3. coronoid process
   4. mandibular foramen
   5. median palatine suture

16. Protection from excessive exposure to radiation is aided by use of aluminum filters and a lead diaphragm. The filters reduce the amount of soft radiation reaching the patient's face and the diaphragm controls the area exposed.
   1. both statements are true
   2. both statements are false
   3. the first statement is true, the second is false
   4. the first statement is false, the second is true

17. Approximately what percent of energy released in the x-ray tube is released as x-rays?
   1. 1%
   2. 10%
   3. 50
   4. 90%
   5. 99%

18. If the temperature of processing solutions is slightly above normal, radiographs of desired density may be best obtained by:
   1. increasing fixing time
   2. decreasing fixing time
   3. increasing developing time
   4. decreasing developing time
   5. increasing exposure time

19. A dental x-ray machine that is set at more than 70 kVp is required to have a total filtration of at least how many millimeters of aluminum?
   1. 1.5
   2. 2.0
   3. 2.5
   4. 3.0
   5. 3.5

20. For x-ray timers calibrated in impulses, how many impulses are there in a second?
   1. 10
   2. 30
   3. 60
   4. 100
   5. 220

21. In taking dental radiographs, the greatest dose of radiation to structures in the patient's jaw comes from:
   1. the primary beam
   2. leakage from the x-ray machine
   3. scatter from the patient's face
   4. scatter from the open-ended position-indicating device

22. The purpose of filtering an x-ray beam is to:
   1. strain out electrons
   2. reduce beam diameter
   3. reduce scatter radiation
   4. remove low energy photons
   5. remove hard penetrating x-rays

23. The time between exposure to x-rays and appearance of radiation damage is the:
   1. silent period
   2. latent period
   3. waiting period
   4. refractory period

24. Ionization has occurred when:
   1. cell death takes place
   2. photons penetrate matter
   3. radiant energy is converted to heat
   4. an electron is displaced from it's orbit

5. an electron is transmitted from the target toward the object

6. all of the above

25. X-rays differ from light in that x-rays:
    1. have more energy
    2. have a greater wavelength
    3. are usually monochromatic
    4. are electromagnetic radiation

26. The energy of photons produced in an x-ray machine is dependent on:
    1. mA
    2. kVp
    3. film type
    4. exposure time
    5. filament temperature

27. Which of the following appears radiopaque in a radiograph?
    1. condensing osteitis
    2. periapical granuloma
    3. apical periodontal cyst
    4. chronic periapical abscess

28. Radiographic changes evident in gingivitis include:
    1. a widened lamina dura
    2. loss of interdental supporting bone
    3. both (1) and (2)
    4. neither (1) nor (2)

29. Factors important in determining the shielding needed for an x-ray unit include all of the following *except:*
    1. operator training
    2. type of x-ray unit
    3. proximity of other workers
    4. composition of existing walls
    5. number of films taken per day

30. Arrange the following cells and tissues from the most sensitive to least sensitive to ionizing radiation:
    a. nerve
    b. bone
    c. lymphocytes
    d. gastrointestinal tract
    1. b,a,d,c
    2. c,a,d,b
    3. c,b,a,d
    4. c,d,a,b
    5. c,d,b,a

31. Arrange the following in order off increasing radiopacity:
    a. dentin
    b. enamel
    c. amalgam

    d. zinc oxide-eugenol
    e. periodontal ligament space
    1. c,b,a,e,d
    2. d,e,c,a,b
    3. e,a,b,d,c,
    4. e,d,a,b,c

32. Which of the following cause film fog in developed radiographs?
    a. underexposure
    b. scattered radiation
    c. improper safelighting
    d. light leak in the dark room
    e. processing solutions that are too cold
    1. a, b, c
    2. a,b,c,d
    3. a,b,e
    4. b,c,d
    5. b,c,d,e
    6. c,d,e

33. Which of the following are needed before dental radiographs are taken?
    a. medical history
    b. clinical examination
    c. history of previous radiographs
    1. a and b
    2. a and c
    3. b and c
    4. all of the above

34. The arrow on the radiograph (Fig. A-7) points to:
    1. mandibular canal
    2. submandibular fossa
    3. buccinator line
    4. internal oblique ridge
    5. external oblique ridge

35. What is the most likely interpretation of the entity indicated by the arrow in Fig. A-8?
    1. root tip
    2. odontoma
    3. microdont
    4. foreign body
    5. osteosclerosis

36. In the radiograph (Fig. A-9) the likely primary cause of the radiolucency at the apex of the second molar is:
    1. dental caries
    2. malignant tumor
    3. developmental
    4. occlusal trauma
    5. internal resorption

Fig. A-7

Fig. A-8

Fig. A-9

Fig. A-10

37. The most probable cause of the error illustrated in Fig. A-10 is:
1. movement of the patient
2. improper vertical angulation
3. improper horizontal angulation
4. use of the paralleling technique
5. use of exhausted processing solutions

38. The entity indicated by the arrow in Fig A-11 is:
1. the zygomatic arch
2. the hamular process
3. a chemical artifact
4. the coronoid process
5. the patient's finger

Fig. A-11

Fig. A-12

39. The technical error in the radiograph (Fig. A-12) is:
1. use of low kVp
2. use of low mAs
3. reversal of film
4. use of outdated film
5. films touching during development

40. Which of the following structures appear radiopaque on a radiograph?
1. mental foramen, genial tubercle, lamina dura
2. external oblique ridge, condyle, anterior nasal spine
3. maxillary sinus, nasal fossa, internal oblique ridge
4. mandibular canal, mylohyoid ridge, nares
5. lamina dura, anterior nasal spine, mandibular foramen

ANSWERS FOR NATIONAL BOARD (NB) QUESTIONS

1.	2	21.	1
2.	3	22.	4
3.	4	23.	2
4.	1	24.	4
5.	4	25.	1
6.	2	26.	2
7.	1	27.	1
8.	2	28.	4
9.	5	29.	1
10.	2	30.	5
11.	3	31.	3
12.	1	32.	4
13.	4	33.	4
14.	1	34.	1
15.	4	35.	1
16.	1	36.	3
17.	1	37.	1
18.	4	38.	4
19.	3	39.	3
20.	3	40.	2

Glossary

administrative radiographs Radiographs taken for other than diagnostic purposes, for example, radiographs taken for verification for third-party payment.

ALARA principle The acronym for "as low as reasonably achievable." In dental radiology, reasonably refers to cost and convenience to the patient.

ala-tragus line An imaginary line between the ala of the nose and the tragus of the ear that is kept parallel to the floor for maxillary periapical and bite-wing films.

alternating current (AC) Electric current that travels in one direction and then reverses its flow to go in the opposite direction.

ampere The unit of measurement of the amount of current flowing in an electric circuit. The unit milliampere (mA) is 1/1000 of an ampere and is the important unit of current measurement pertaining to an x-ray tube.

Angstrom unit (A) A unit of measurement equal to 1/100,000,000 cm; x-ray wavelengths are expressed in Angstrom units.

anode The positive charged side of the dental x-ray tube. It contains the tungsten target at which the electrons are aimed and from which x-rays are emitted.

atom The basic unit of matter, composed of a positively charged nucleus around which negative electrons revolve.

atomic number The number of protons in the nucleus of an atom. Its symbol is Z and is written as the subscript, for example, $_3$Li.

attenuation Absorbing or weakening of an x-ray beam because of passage through a material.

autotransformer A transformer that has only one coil and a series of taps that allows it to step up or step down voltage.

background radiation The ever-present ionizing radiation in the environment. Its sources included cosmic rays, radioactive materials, industrial waste and nuclear fallout.

barrier A radiation-absorbing material such as lead, concrete, or plaster used to protect the area from radiation.

bequerel The Systeme Internationale (SI) unit of radioactivity produced by the disintegration of unstable elements. It replaces the curie.

binding The energy expressed in electron volts that binds the orbiting electrons in their respective shell around the nucleus of an atom.

bisecting-angle technique A technique for intraoral periapical radiography where the film packet is positioned as close to tooth and bone as possible and the central x-ray is directed vertically at an imaginary line that bisects the angle formed by the long axis of the tooth and the film packet.

bite-wing radiographs Intraoral films that show only the crown portions of opposing teeth in the biting position.

bremsstrahlung The release of a photon of energy by a bombarding electron slowed and bent off course by an atom.

buccal object rule In localization if the object moves relatively on a second radiograph in the opposite direction as the horizontal tube shift, then the object is buccally positioned.

calcium tungstate The fluorescent material used to coat intensifying screens.

cassette A wrapping or container for x-ray film that is light-tight and will permit penetration of x-rays. Cassettes may be plastic, card board, or metal.

cathode The negatively charged side of the dental x-ray tube. It contains the tungsten filament and the molybdenum focusing cup.

cathode ray The stream of electrons in the x-ray tube traveling from filament to target.

central ray That x-ray that is located in the center of the x-ray beam as it leaves the tube head.

cephalometric radiograph The process of measuring the skull by means of radiographs.

cervical burnout The shadow seen interproximally on radiographs that is caused by the concavity in the root surface at that area. It may resemble caries.

characteristic x-rays X-rays that are produced when orbiting electrons in an atom fall from outer shells to inner shells after an orbiting electron is knocked out of one of the inner shells by bombarding electrons.

chromosomes One of a definite number of rod like bodies, containing genes, found in the nucleus of a cell. At the time of cell division they divide and distribute evenly in the resulting cells.

collimation The process of restricting the size of the x-ray beam.

collimator A device that limits the size of the x-ray beam.

computed tomography (CT) (CAT scan) Tomographic process in which x-ray scanning produces digital data that measure the extent of the energy transmission through an object. This information is stored and transformed by a computer into a density scale that is used to generate an image.

cone The pointed PID on the dental x-ray machine through which the x-rays travel after leaving the tube.

cone cutting The mistake made by not centering the x-ray beam on the film, leading to unexposed areas on the film.

contrast The difference in densities between adjacent areas on the radiograph.

cosmic ray A radiation that has its origin outside of the earth's atmosphere, for example, the sun's rays.

curie The unit of measurement of the number of nuclear disintegrations of a radioactive element. The curie was replaced by the becquerel in 1985.

cycle of electric current The sine wave plot of the change in polarity of an alternating current circuit where the current travels first in the positive direction and then in the negative direction.

definition or detail The degree of clarity on a radiograph.

density (film) The degree of blackness on a radiograph.

density (object) The relative mass of an object through which x-ray beam passes, which makes it appear radiopaque or radiolucent.

dent program (dental exposure normalization technique) An exposure reduction and quality assurance program for radiological health agencies developed by the Federal Center for Devices and Radiological Health.

developer The solution used in the processing of exposed x-ray film that precipitates silver from the silver bromide crystals of the film emulsion that have been energized by x-rays.

developer cutoff The blank area on processed radiographs that results from an insufficient

level of solution in the developer tank in the darkroom.

diaphragm The lead doughnut-shaped collimating device found in the dental x-ray machine that limits the beam size.

dimensional distortion The distortion seen in the bisecting-angle technique when parts of the object farther from the film are foreshortened in relation to parts of the object closer to the film, for example, buccal roots of maxillary molars versus palatal root.

direct current (DC) Electric current that flows in one direction and does not reverse itself.

dose The amount of radiation energy absorbed per unit mass of tissue at a particular site.

dose equivalent A concept that allows for the fact that not all radiations are identical in biologic effects. The dose equivalent is expressed in rems or sieverts.

duty cycle The number of seconds in a minute that a dental x-ray machine can be operated without overheating.

duty rating The number of consecutive seconds that a dental x-ray machine can be operated before overheating.

electric current The flow of electricity through a circuit.

electromagnetic radiation spectrum A group of energy-bearing invisible radiations whose individual properties are determined by their wavelengths. X-rays are electromagnetic radiations.

electron A negatively charged particle, which is a constituent of every neutral atom.

electrostatic imaging An imaging technique in which a charged plate is used as the receptor, as in xeroradiography.

elongation The distortion on a radiograph that results in lengthening of the image.

emulsion The silver halide suspension in gelatin that is coated on the x-ray film base.

exposure A measure of the ionization in air produced by x or gamma radiation.

exposure time The amount of time, expressed in seconds or impulses, that x-rays are generated.

extension paralleling technique A technique for intraoral radiography that uses a 16-inch focal-film distance and film packet placement parallel to the long axis of the teeth and a central ray direction perpendicular to both object and film.

extraoral films Radiographs that are taken with the film outside the patient's mouth.

fallout A form of background radiation produced by nuclear explosions.

filament The tungsten wire found at the cathode in the x-ray tube, which when heated will boil off electrons.

film badge A recording device worn to record one's exposure to ionizing radiation.

film reversal The improper placement of the film packet in the patient's mouth, which results in an underexposed film with geometric images (herringbone pattern) on it, caused by the useful beam striking the lead foil backing before the film.

film speed or sensitivity An expression of how much radiation for what period of time (mAs) will be necessary to produce an image on the film.

filter An aluminum disk placed in the path of the useful beam, which absorbs the softer, less penetrating radiations.

fixer The solution used in the processing of exposed x-ray film that removes the unaffected silver bromide crystals from the emulsion and preserves the image.

fluorescence The property of emitting visible light when struck by radiation.

focal-film distance (FFD) The distance from the focal spot (target) at the anode of the dental x-ray tube to the film. It is usually expressed in inches (e.g., 8-inch FFD).

focal spot See *target*.

focal trough That plane of an object that is seen clearly on a laminograph.

fog A detrimental density imparted to radiographic image by the film base and chemical action on unexposed silver grains. Fog is increased by inadvertent exposure to white light or a poor safelight.

foreshortening The distortion on a radiograph that results in shortening of the image.

full-mouth survey A series of intraoral radiographs that gives diagnostic information for all teeth and desired bony areas. It is usually composed of periapical and bite-wing films.

gag reflex The retching, coughing, or vomiting caused by contact of the film packet, holding device, or operator's fingers with the patient's palate or other intraoral tissues.

gamma rays Radiations that emanate from radioactive materials.

gene The basic unit of inheritance located in the chromosome; it determines hereditary characteristics.

genetic effects The changes produced in an individual's genes and chromosomes; usually refers to those changes in reproductive cells.

gray (gy) The Systeme Internationale unit for absorbed dose. One gray equals 100 rads.

H & D curve The H & D (Hurter and Driffield) curve is a plot that shows the relationship be-

tween film exposure and its resultant density.

half-value layer The thickness of a specific material that attenuates the x-ray beam intensity to one half. It is an expression of beam quality.

horizontal angulation The aiming of the x-ray, beam in the horizontal plane.

image receptor The film, xeroradiographic plate, or film screen combination that the x-rays strike to produce the visible image.

intensifying screen A coating of fluorescent material on a suitable base that will intensify the radiation, thus permitting a decrease in exposure time.

inverse-square law An expression of the relationship between the exposure time and the focal-film distance. It states that the intensity of the radiation varies inversely to the square of the distance.

ion An electrically charged (+ or −) particle of matter.

ionization The process by which an electrically stable or neutral atom or molecule gains or loses electrons and thereby acquires either a positive or negative charge.

ionizing radiation The property of radiation that produces ions when interacting with matter.

isotopes Atoms whose nuclei have the same number of protons but a different number of neutrons.

kilovolt One thousand volts.

kilovolt peak (kVp) Used in dental radiology to describe the kilovoltage setting on the control panel. It implies that not all the x-rays generated will be of the penetrating power called for; rather the numerical setting will be the peak.

labial mounting A means of mounting and viewing processed radiographs so that the observer is looking into the patient's mouth with the patient's right side on the viewer's left.

laminogram A radiograph of a three dimensional object that shows a predetermined plane clearly while blurring out all other superimposed structures.

latent image The term used to describe the x-ray film after it has been exposed. The film contains the latent image that will be made visible by the film processing.

latent period The delay between exposure of an organism to radiation and manifestation of change produced by that radiation.

lingual mounting A means of mounting and viewing processed radiographs so that the observer seems to be looking at the teeth from within the patient's mouth with the patient's right side on the viewer's right.

localized exposure The measurement of radiation to the area of the body that is in the path of the direct beam of radiation.

long cone Used to refer to cones on x-ray machines where focal-film distance is 16 inches or greater.

magnetic resonance imaging (MRI) An imaging technique that uses magnetic fields and radio-frequencies to produce computed tomographic sections of the body.

mass number The number of nucleons (protons and neutrons) in the nucleus of an atom.

milliampere (mA) One one-thousandth (1/1000) of an ampere.

milliroentgen (mR) One one-thousandth (1/1000) of a roentgen.

molecule The smallest particle of a substance that retains the properties of the substance.

mutation The chemical effect of a change in a gene or a chromosomal aberration.

neutron A particle that has no charge but has mass. It is found in the nucleus of an atom.

nucleus The positively charged, relatively heavy inner core of an atom.

object The structure being radiographed, such as tooth or bone.

object-film distance The distance between the object and the x-ray film.

occlusal film A large piece of intraoral film that is placed on the occlusal surfaces of either upper or lower teeth and used to portray objects in the third dimension.

orbit A prescribed path or ring that electrons travel in around the nucleus of an atom.

output The amount of radiation being produced by the x-ray machine. It is measured in roentgens per second.

packet A wrapping or container for intraoral x-ray film that is light-tight and will permit penetration of x-rays. Packets are usually made of paper or cardboard.

panoramic film A radiograph that shows both the mandible and the maxilla in their entirety.

pantomogram A panoramic radiograph taken made by using curved surface tomography.

paralleling technique A technique for intraoral of an periapical radiography in which the film of packet is positioned parallel to the long axis of the tooth and the central ray is directed perpendicular to both tooth and film packet.

penetration The ability of x-rays to pass through an object and reach the film.

penumbra The amount of unsharpness of the image.

periapical radiograph An intraoral film that shows the entire tooth and surrounding bony structures.

photon A discrete unit of energy.

point of entry Anatomic location on the patient's face at which the central x-ray is aimed so that the x-rays will strike the center of the film in the patient's mouth.

position-indicating device (PID) That part of the x-ray machine (cone, rectangle, or cylinder) that aligns the useful beam to the object and film.

primary radiation X-rays coming directly from the target of the x-ray tube.

progeny The descendants of an individual.

proton The positively charged particle that has mass. It is found in the nucleus of an atom.

quality assurance A series of tests and procedures to ensure that all components of the radiographic system are functioning at an acceptable level of quality and thus to ensure the best radiograph for the radiation exposure.

radiation The emission and propagation of energy in the forms of waves or particles.

radiation absorbed dose (rad) A unit of absorbed radiation equal to 100 ergs per gram. In dental radiology a rad is approximately equal to a roentgen.

radiation exposure The process of being struck by radiation, either primary or secondary.

radiograph The visual image produced by chemically processing the effects of x-rays on film.

radiolucent The black areas on radiographs.

radiopaque The white areas on radiographs.

receptor The material (film, film screen, or xeroradiographic charged plate) that is affected by the x-ray beam and from which the visible image is formed.

receptor holder The device that holds and positions the receptor (e.g., film) in the patient's mouth.

rectangular collimation Limiting the shape of an x-ray beam to a rectangle instead of the conventional circle.

rectification The blocking of the flow of current in one direction in an alternating current circuit.

reference film An ideally processed film, which is kept on the darkroom viewbox, to which densities can be compared to check processing solutions.

right-angle technique See *Paralleling technique*.

roentgen The basic unit for measuring x-ray (ionizing radiation) exposure in air. It is the amount of radiation needed to produce one electrostatic charge in 1 cubic centimeter of air. The milliroentgen (mR) is 1/1000 of a roentgen (R).

roentgen equivalent man (rem) The expression of dose equivalent; the dose of radiation that will produce the same biologic effects in humans as are produced by 1 roentgen of x-radiation. For x-rays the rem equals the rad.

safelight Illumination used in the darkroom that will not affect the film emulsion.

sagittal plane of head A median vertical longitudinal plane that divides the head into right and left halves.

scattered radiation Radiation that during its passage through a substance has been deviated in direction. It may also have been modified by an increase in wavelength. It is one form of secondary radiation.

secondary radiation Radiation that comes from any matter being struck by primary radiation. Secondary x-rays are less penetrating than primary x-rays.

selection criteria Those factors that determine whether radiographs are necessary and useful in a specific clinical situation.

shielding Preventing or reducing the passage of radiation particles.

short cone A term used to refer to cones on dental x-ray machines where focal-film distance is 8 inches.

sievert (SV) The Systeme Internationale unit for the dose equivalent. One sievert equals 100 rem.

sight development An unacceptable technique used to process x-ray films. The time the film stays in the developer is determined by periodically looking at the developing image under safelight conditions.

silver bromides The x-ray-sensitive crystals that are used in the film emulsion.

soft x-rays X-rays of longer wavelengths that have low penetration.

somatic effects Effects of radiation on all cells except the reproductive cells.

systems internationale units The units of radiation measurement that standardize measurement to the metric system.

target That part of the anode that the high speed electrons strike and that produces x-rays and heat. In dental x-ray tubes, the target is usually made of tungsten.

thermionic emission effect The production of free electrons by passing an electric current through a tungsten filament and thus heating the filament.

time-temperature development A technique used to process x-ray films where the time the film stays in the developer is related to the temperature of the solution within a stated acceptable temperature range.

tissue sensitivity That scale of sensitivity of various tissues in the body to radiations. Some tissues (e.g., epithelium) are very radiosensitive, while others (e.g., bone) are relatively radioresistant.

tomograph See *Laminogram.*

total body exposure The radiation dosage that reflects the effects on the whole body of the person exposed.

transformer An electric device that can either increase (step up) or decrease (step down) voltage.

ultrasound Sound wavelengths used for diagnostic imaging that lies above the audible range.

useful beam The part of the primary radiation that passes through the diaphragm aperture and filter and exits through the PID.

vertical angulation The angle made between the x-ray beam and a line parallel to the floor.

voltage The difference in potential in an electric circuit. It is this difference that causes the current to flow.

wavelength The distance from the crest of one wave to the crest of the next wave. The length of the wave determines its energy.

xeroradiography An imaging system that uses a charged plate as the receptor. The images are then printed by the xerographic copying process.

x-rays Penetrating electromagnetic radiations having wavelengths shorter than those of visible light, which are produced by bombarding a metal target with high-speed electrons.

Index